C. Heiligensetzer
S. Buchfink
H.-J. Herschlein
M. Huber
A. Schaffert
R. R. Zink

ENGLISH
DEUTSCH
FARSI
فارسی

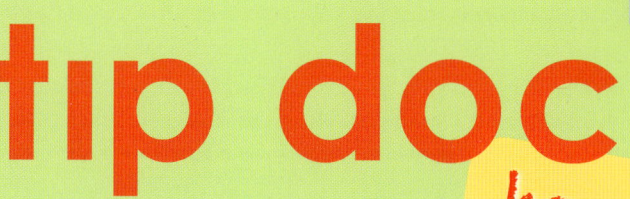

گفتگوی پزشک و بیمار با تصویر
Arzt-Patient-Gespräch in Bildern
The doctor-patient-discussion in pictures

Christina Heiligensetzer (Herausgeberin)
tıp doc home – Arzt-Patient-Gespräch in Bildern, englisch – deutsch – farsi

Autoren: Dr. med. Christina Heiligensetzer (Fachärztin für Urologie) – Unter Mitarbeit von: Safiye Buchfink (Zahnärztin), Prof. Dr. med. Hans-Joachim Herschlein (Facharzt für Gynäkologie), Dr. med. Meike Huber (Fachärztin für Pädiatrie), Dr. med. Andreas Schaffert (Facharzt für Allgemeinmedizin), Dr. med. René R. Zink (Facharzt für Orthopädie) – **Übersetzung:** Mohammad Davoudi, John Castner, Bild und Sprache e. V. **Bildgebung:** Alf Setzer und Christina Heiligensetzer – **Buchgestaltung:** Eva Knoll, Stuttgart

Lieber Leser – die Medizin unterliegt heutzutage einem ständigen Wandel. Die Autoren haben mit großer Gewissenhaftigkeit geprüft, dass die in diesem Werk gemachten Angaben dem heutigen Wissensstand und den Erfordernissen der Medizin entsprechen. Dennoch entbindet dies den Nutzer nicht von der Pflicht, anhand der Beipackzettel, der aktuellen medizinischen Veröffentlichungen und von Wörterbüchern die Angaben zu überprüfen und Rücksprache mit seinem behandelnden Arzt resp. mit einem Spezialisten oder Dolmetscher zu halten. Die Verordnung und Einnahme geschieht in eigener Verantwortung.

Dear reader – we have carefully edited all of the information in this book. Nevertheless, in case of problems understanding the text, please consider the help of an interpreter. We are not responsible for incorrect treatment, therapies and applications due to the use of this book in any case.

خواننده گرامی - امروزه پزشکی همواره شاهد دگرگونی است . این کتاب با دقت کامل نویسندگان بررسی شده است تا اطلاعات آن با آخرین یافته های پزشکی همخوانی داشته باشد. با این وجود خواننده این کتاب باید با کمک دفترچه راهنمای همراه دارو، یافته های جدید پزشکی ولغتنامه ها این اطلاعات و ترجمه ها را دوباره کنترل کند و با پزشک خود و یا مترجم در میان بگذارد.

Dieses Werk und alle seine Teile sind urheberrechtlich geschützt. Die Verwertung der Texte und Bilder, Photographien und Graphiken, Nachdruck, Vervielfältigungen in jeder Form, Speicherung, Sendung oder Übertragung des Werks ganz oder teilweise auf Papier oder die Verarbeitung mit elektronischen Systemen wie Film, Daten- oder Tonträgern einschließlich zukünftiger Medien sind ohne Zustimmung des Verlags unzulässig und strafbar. Dies gilt auch für Übersetzungen und Übertragungen in andere Sprachen und Länder.

© setzer verlag, 2010
alf setzer, seyfferstraße 53, 70197 stuttgart
www.setzer-verlag.de, info@setzer-verlag.de
ISBN 978-3-9813673-2-4

Contents	Inhalt	موضوع	
FAQ	Häufige Fragen	سوالهای معمول	A
Numbers and times	Zahlen und Zeiten	عددها و زمانها	B
Questionnaire	Fragebogen	پرسشنامه	8
At the reception	An der Anmeldung	هنگام پذیرش	11
At the family doctor	Beim Hausarzt	پیش پزشک خانواده	12
Organs	Organe	اعضای بدن	22
At the pediatrician	Beim Kinderarzt	پیش پزشک کودکان	25
At the gynecologist	Beim Frauenarzt	پیش پزشک زنان	32
Pregnancy	Schwangerschaft	حاملگی	40
At the urologist	Beim Urologen	پیش متخصص اورلوژی	U2
At the orthopedist	Beim Orthopäden	پیش متخصص ارتوپدی	42
At the dentist	Beim Zahnarzt	پیش دندانپزشک	46
Examination	Untersuchung	معاینه	49
Treatment	Behandlung	درمان	54
Nutrition	Ernährung	تغذیه	63
At the hospital	Im Krankenhaus	در بیمارستان	68
Nursing	Pflege	پرستاری	70
In the pharmacy	In der Apotheke	در داروخانه	76
Traveler´s health kit	Reiseapotheke	داروخانه مسافرت	77
Index	Stichwortverzeichnis	فهرست کلمات کلیدی	79

Thank you very much!   Wir sagen DANKE   سپاسگذاری

Brad Alexander, Stuttgart
Quynh Bach, Stuttgart
Erika Binder, Fachärztin für Gynäkologie, Stuttgart
Karrol Castner, Las Vegas
John Castner, New York
Mohammad Davoudi, Darmstadt
Dr. med. Yadollah Davoudi, Facharzt für Urologie, Wuppertal
Emil, Emma, Marlene und Wendelin, Stuttgart
Peter Forstmann, Reeseberg-Apotheke, Hamburg
Mathilde Heiligensetzer, Betzigau
Prof. Dr. Katrin Höhmann, Pädagogische Hochschule, Ludwigsburg
Jing Li, Langenbach
Ortema GmbH, Orthopädietechnik, Waiblingen/Markgröningen
WiVa Med, Praxis für Physiotherapie, Waiblingen
insbesondere
Stabsstelle des Integrationsbeauftragten der Landesregierung Baden-Württemberg
Bild und Sprache e. V.

und viele andere

Vocabulary   Vokabeln   کلمه ها

yes	ja	بله
no	nein	نه
please	bitte	لطفا
thank you	danke	مرسی
I´m sorry!	Entschuldigung!	ببخشید!
My name is …	Ich heiße …	اسم من ... هست.
What´s your name?	Wie heißen Sie?	اسم شما چیست؟
How are you?	Wie geht es Ihnen?	حال شما چطور است؟
Good morning!	Guten Morgen!	صبح بخیر!
Good afternoon! (>12.00)	Guten Tag!	روز بخیر!
Good night!	Gute Nacht!	شب بخیر!
Good-bye!	Auf Wiedersehen!	خداحافظ!
I don´t want.	Ich will/möchte nicht.	نمیخواهم.
I can´t.	Ich kann nicht.	نمیتوانم.

| Preface | Einführung | مقدمه |

خواننده گرامی،

ما پزشکان سالهای زیادی از این موضوع ناخشنود بودیم که نمیتوانستیم با بیماران خارجی به خوبی ارتباط برقرار کنیم. راههای ترجمه موثری پیدا نکردیم و به همین خاطر شروع به کشیدن تصویر کردیم تا این کتاب به وجود آمد.

تقسیم بندی متن بوسیله رنگها با فهرست به فهمیدن سریعتر کمک میکند. برای ما مهم بود کلمات را طوری دسته بندی کنیم که معمولا مرتبط با هم در صحبت با بیمار پیش می آید. صفحه های آ و ب با سوالهای معمول و عددها و زمانها قابل جدا شدن هستند تا بتوان آنها را کنار صفحات دیگر گذاشت. با ضمیمه کردن متن میتوان مطمئن بود که برای همه تصویر و ترجمه آن به سرعت قابل فهم است. در دفترچه های جداگانه برای بیماران اطلاعاتی در مورد زنان و ارولوژی به زبانهای مختلف در سایت اینترنتی ما موجود است.

این کتاب جایگزین آماده کردن ذهنی بیمار توسط پزشک برای عمل جراحی نیست و ما همچنین در این کتاب از توضیح سرطان صرف نظر کردیم چون در این موارد احتیاج به یک مترجم با سابقه داریم.

این کتاب نتیجه تلاش یک مجموعه خصوصی است که با استفاده از تجربیات انسانهای زیادی به راه خود ادامه میدهد. بنابراین در چاپ دوم این کتاب به خاطر پیشنهادات شما تعداد زیادی از کلمات جدید آورده شده است. ما ادعای کامل بودن نداریم و همیشه از نظرات شما استقبال میکنیم. اگر شما به کلمات دیگری احتیاج دارید و یا ایده جدیدی دارید با آدرس زیرتماس بگیرید.
www.medi-bild.de با آرزوی بهبود و سلامت برای همه بیماران.
به امید اینکه بتوانیم همدیگر را بهتر بفهمیم.

نویسندگان

Preface — Einführung — مقدمه

Lieber Leser,

über Jahre hinweg waren wir unzufrieden, dass wir als Ärzte uns mit unseren fremdsprachigen Patienten oft nicht ausreichend verständigen konnten. Funktionierende Übersetzungshilfen für die Praxis haben wir nicht gefunden. Darum nahmen wir den Zeichenstift selbst in die Hand. Entstanden ist dieses Buch.

Die farbige Gliederung und Querverweise helfen dabei, sich schnell zu verständigen. Im Interesse einer höchstmöglichen Praktikabilität haben wir uns bemüht, die Begriffe so zu gruppieren, wie sie im Patientengespräch häufig zusammenhängend vorkommen. Seite A und B mit *Häufigen Fragen* und *Zahlen und Zeiten* sind zum Heraustrennen, damit man sie neben jede andere Seite legen kann. Durch knappe Untertitel ist sichergestellt, dass alle den Sinn eines Bildes und der Übersetzung in Sekundenschnelle erfassen können. Das Kapitel Urologie ist gesondert in einem Begleitheft erschienen.

Das Buch ersetzt nicht das Aufklärungsgespräch vor Operationen. Ebenso haben wir auf die Aufklärung einer Krebskrankheit verzichtet. Für diese Gespräche halten wir die Hilfe eines geschulten Dolmetschers für unersetzbar.

Dieses Buch ist das Ergebnis einer Privatinitiative, die davon lebt, dass viele Menschen ihre Erfahrungen einbringen. So haben wir in der 2. Auflage auf Ihre Wünsche hin viele neue Begriffe eingearbeitet. Wir erheben keinen Anspruch auf Perfektion und freuen uns immer über Anregungen. Wenn Sie weitere Vokabeln benötigen oder Ideen haben, wenden Sie sich gerne an uns oder den Verein *Bild und Sprache e. V.*, der die weiteren Begriffe und aktuelle Materialien auf seiner Seite www.medi-bild.de zum Download bereit hält.

Nun wünschen wir unseren und allen Patienten baldige Genesung, Gesundheit, und dass wir uns gut verstehen.

Die Autoren

| symbols:
Symbole:
 | 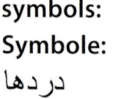 pain
Schmerzen
دردها | 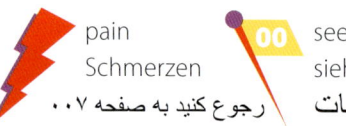 see page 00
siehe Seite 00
رجوع کنید به صفحه ۰۰۷ | ~xyz word repetition
Wortwiederholung
نشانه: تکرار کلمات |

Preface   Einführung   مقدمه

Dear reader,

over the years we have been dissatisfied that there was no proper translation of our book available to foreign-language speaking patients. Efficient translation aids were not on hand. So we took up the pencil ourselves to provide you with our information in this book.

Each chapter addresses specific issues and keeps in mind the daily practices of our respective target readers, and is therefore not dependent on medical classifications and terms. Colored diagrams with cross-references and explanations will help you to quickly and easily understand the information. Short phrases that are to the point, make sure that everybody is able to understand within seconds the idea of the picture and its interpretation. The chapter urology was released in an extra journal. The detachable pages A and B with *FAQ* and *Numbers and times* could be laid right beside their respective page and all the information will line up. This book is no substitution for the pre-operation discussion or the disclosure of having cancer. In our opinion, these patient-doctor discussions need the help of an interpreter and are not replaceable.

This book grew out of a private initiative which brings in the experience of many people. We do not claim perfection. If you have other phrases or more ideas, feel free to contact us or the association *Bild und Sprache e. V.*. On their webside www.medi-pic.com you will find more material and topical issues (e. g. the questionnaire) for free download.

We wish all of our patients, and all other patients as well, a speedy recovery, health and a good understanding.

The Authors

Please fill in the attached questionnaire and take it with you to your medical appointment. Be so kind and answer all questions completely, regardless of whether you consider them important for your current problem or not.

Füllen Sie umseitigen Fragebogen bitte aus und bringen Sie ihn zu Ihrem Arztbesuch mit. Beantworten Sie bitte alle Fragen vollständig, egal, ob Sie es für Ihr aktuelles Problem für wichtig erachten oder nicht.

لطفا پرسشنامه پشت این صفحه را پر کنید و آن را به پزشک خود نشان دهید. به تمام سوالها به طور کامل جواب دهید صرف نظر از اینکه این سوالها را برای مشکل خود مهم میدانید یا نه.

Vor dem Arztbesuch
Fragebogen

قبل از دیدار با پزشک
پرسشنامه

01. Name .... نام و نام خانوادگی	e-mail .... پست الکترونیک .١
Familienstand .... وضعیت تاهل	Telefon .... تلفن/ همراه
Beruf/Firma .... شغل/ محل کار	Kinder .... فرزند

02. Bitte schildern Sie Ihre jetzigen Beschwerden! — ٢. لطفا بیماری خود را توضیح دهید.

....

03. Welche anderen Krankheiten haben Sie (siehe Liste)? — ٣. چه بیماریهای دیگری دارید؟ (رجوع کنید به پائین)

04. Welche Operationen hatten Sie (siehe auch Liste)? — ٤. چه عمل جراحی تا به حال داشته اید؟ (رجوع کنید به پائین)

- ☐ Schlaganfall • مغز   ☐ Bluthochdruck • فشار خون   ☐ Herz • قلب
- ☐ Schilddrüse • غده تیروئید   ☐ Zucker • مرض قند   ☐ Thrombose • لخته خونی دررگ
- ☐ Hepatitis • هپاتیت   ☐ Leber • کبد   ☐ Galle • کیسه صفرا   ☐ Magen • معده
- ☐ Brust • سینه   ☐ Hämorrhoiden • بواسیر   ☐ Blinddarm • آپاندیس   ☐ Darm • روده
- ☐ Kaiserschnitt • سزارین   ☐ Ausschabung • کورتاژ   ☐ Gebärmutter • رحم
- ☐ Lunge • ریه   ☐ Prostata • غده پروستات   ☐ Blase • مثانه   ☐ Niere • کلیه
- ☐ Knochen • استخوانها   ☐ Muskeln • ماهیچه ها   ☐ Nerven • اعصاب   ☐ Asthma • آسم
- ☐ Arthrose • آرتوروز   ☐ Gelenke • مفاصل   ☐ Wirbelsäule • ستون فقرات
- ☐ Augen • چشم   ☐ Haut • پوست   ☐ Knochenbruch • شکستگی استخوان   ☐ Rheuma • رماتیسم
- ☐ andere • دیگر   ☐ Chemotherapie • شیمی درمانی   ☐ Bestrahlung • اشعه درمانی   ☐ Tumor • غده

05. Welche Medikamente nehmen Sie derzeit? — ۵. در حال حاضر چه داروهایی مصرف میکنید؟

....

06. Sind bei Ihnen Allergien bekannt? — ۶. به چه چیزهائی حساسیت دارید؟
- Medikamente .... دارو   ☐ Nahrungsmittel .... مواد غذائی ☐
- Pollen .... گرده شکوفه   ☐ andere .... دیگر ☐

07. Neigen Sie zu   ☐ Durchfall • اسهال دارید؟   ☐ Verstopfung • ٧. آیا شما مشکل یبوست
08. Körpergewicht kg • کیلو .... وزن   Körpergröße cm .... سانتیمتر ٨. قد
   Gewichtsverlust kg • کیلو .... کاهش وزن؟   Gewichtszunahme kg • کیلو .... افزایش وزن؟
   Seit wann? — ازکی؟ (ازچه وقت؟)
09. Rauchen Sie? .... سیگار میکشید؟   Wie viel? .... ٩. چقدر؟
10. Wie viel Alkohol trinken Sie? .... ١٠. چقدر الکل مینوشید؟

11. Welche Impfungen haben Sie? — ١١. چه واکسنهائی تا به حال زده اید؟
   اگر دفترچه واکسن پیشگیری دارید، همراه خود بیاورید!
   Impfpass – Vorsorgeheft – Bringen Sie es mit!

....

12. — ١٢. آیا در خانواده شما بیماریهای ارثی، غدد و یا متا بولیسمی (مثل مرض قند) وجود دارد؟
   Gibt es Erb-, Tumor- oder Stoffwechselkrankheiten (z. B. Zucker) in der Familie?

....

Before the appointment
Questionnaire

Vor dem Arztbesuch
Fragebogen

01. Name • Name .... e-mail. ....
   marital status • Familienstand .... tel./mobile/Handy ....
   job/company name • Beruf/Firma .... children • Kinder ....

02. Please describe your present problems! • Bitte schildern Sie Ihre jetzigen Beschwerden!
   ....

03. Which other diseases do you have (see list below)? • Welche anderen Krankheiten haben Sie (s. u.)?
   ....

04. What operations have you had (see list below)? • Welche Operationen hatten Sie (siehe auch Liste)?
   ....

- ❏ heart • Herz   ❏ stroke • Schlaganfall   ❏ high blood pressure • Bluthochdruck
- ❏ thrombosis • Thrombose   ❏ diabetes • Zucker   ❏ thyroid gland • Schilddrüse
- ❏ stomach • Magen   ❏ gall bladder • Galle   ❏ liver • Leber   ❏ hepatitis • Hepatitis
- ❏ bowel • Darm   ❏ appendicitis • Blinddarm   ❏ haemorrhoids • Hämorrhoiden   ❏ breast • Brust
- ❏ womb • Gebärmutter   ❏ abrasio • Ausschabung   ❏ cesarean • Kaiserschnitt   ❏ kidney • Niere
- ❏ bladder • Blase   ❏ prostate • Prostata   ❏ lung • Lunge   ❏ asthma • Asthma
- ❏ bronchitis • Bronchitis   ❏ nerves • Nerven   ❏ muscles • Muskeln   ❏ bones • Knochen
- ❏ spine • Wirbelsäule   ❏ joints • Gelenke   ❏ arthrosis • Arthrose   ❏ rheumatism • Rheuma
- ❏ skin • Haut   ❏ eyes • Augen   ❏ tumor • Tumor   ❏ radiation • Bestrahlung
- ❏ chemotherapy • Chemotherapie

05. What medications do you take at present? • Welche Medikamente nehmen Sie derzeit?
   ....

06. Are you aware of any allergies? • Sind bei Ihnen Allergien bekannt?
   ❏ drugs • Medikamente ....   ❏ foods • Nahrungsmittel ....
   ❏ pollen • Pollen ....   ❏ others • andere ....

07. Do you tend to • Neigen Sie zu   ❏ constipation • Verstopfung   ❏ diarrhoea • Durchfall?

08. weight • Körpergewicht .... kg   height • Körpergröße .... cm
   Any loss in weight? • Gewichtsverlust .... kg   Any increase in weight? • -zunahme .... kg
   Since when? • Seit wann? ....

09. Do you smoke? • Rauchen Sie? ....   How much? • Wie viel? ....

10. How much alcohol do you drink?? • Wie viel Alkohol trinken Sie? ....

11. Which inoculations have you had? • Welche Impfungen haben Sie? Vaccination Certificate • Impfpass – Preventive check-up card • Vorsorgeheft – Please bring it! • Bringen Sie es mit!
   ....

12. Are there hereditary, tumor or metabolism (e. g. diabetes) diseases in your family? • Gibt es Erb-, Tumor- oder Stoffwechselkrankheiten (z. B. Zucker) in der Familie?

At the doctor **Beim Arzt** پیش پزشک خانواده

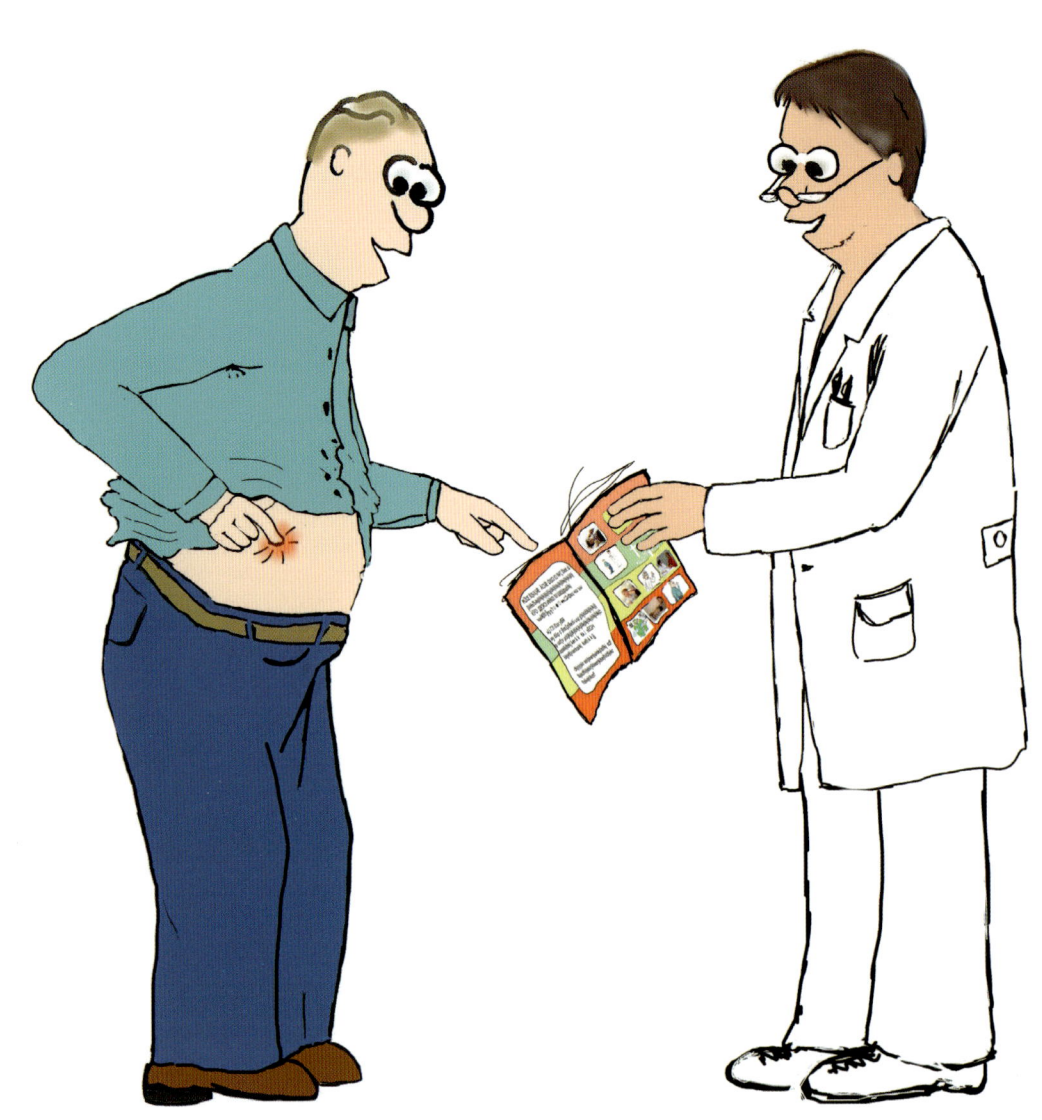

„My problems are here."
Reflect which problems you like to tell the doctor and mark the suitable pictures. Then point on „your" pictures at the doctor´s.

„Ich habe dort Probleme."
Überlegen Sie, welche Beschwerden Sie dem Arzt schildern möchten, und markieren Sie die passenden Bilder. Tippen Sie dann beim Arzt auf „Ihre" Bilder.

„اینجا مشکل دارم."
خوب فکر کنید، کدام بیماری را میخواهید به پزشک توضیح دهید و تصاویر مرتبط را علامت بزنید. هنگام معاینه آنها را به پزشک نشان دهید.

At the reception — An der Anmeldung — هنگام پذیرش

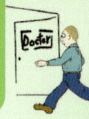

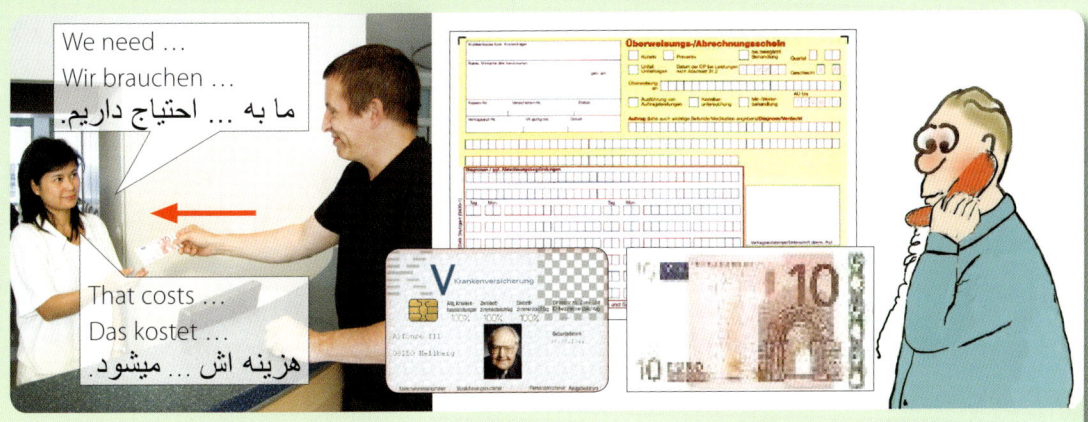

health insurance card	uput	10 €/money	Phone us!
Versicherungskarte	Überweisung	10 €/Geld	Rufen Sie an!
کارت بیمه	حواله	۱۰ یورو/پول	تلفن بزنید!

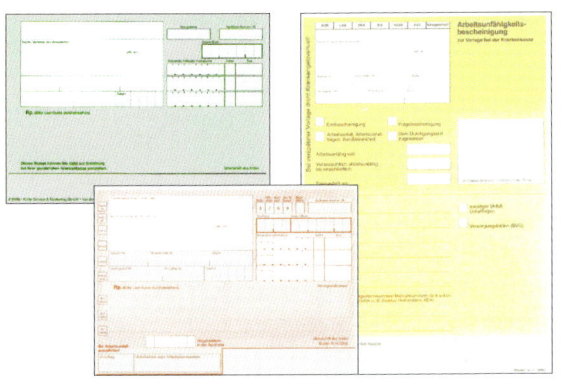

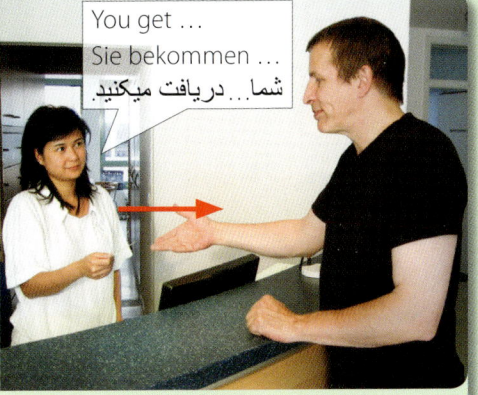

prescription	insurance/private	sick report	examination
Rezept	Kasse/privat	Krankmeldung	Untersuchung
نسخه	خصوصی / نسخه صندوق	گواهی بیماری	معاینه

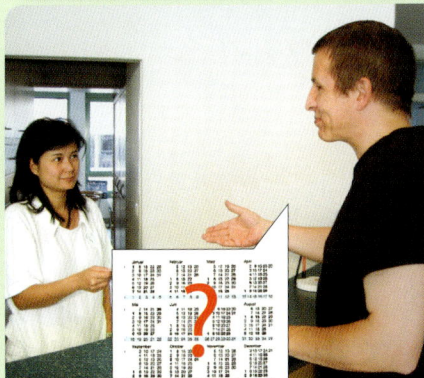

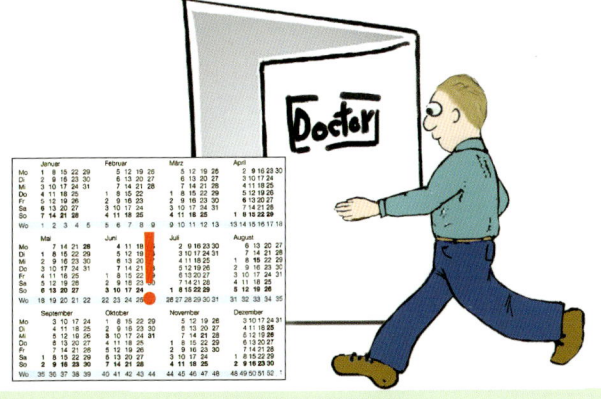

I need an appointment. — Ich brauche einen Termin. — من یک وقت ملاقات میخواهم.

Your next appointment is on the …. — Ihr nächster Termin ist am …. — وقت ملاقات بعدی شما ....

At the family doctor	Beim Hausarzt	پیش پزشک خانواده
Infection/allergies	Infektion/Allergie	سرایت / حساسیت

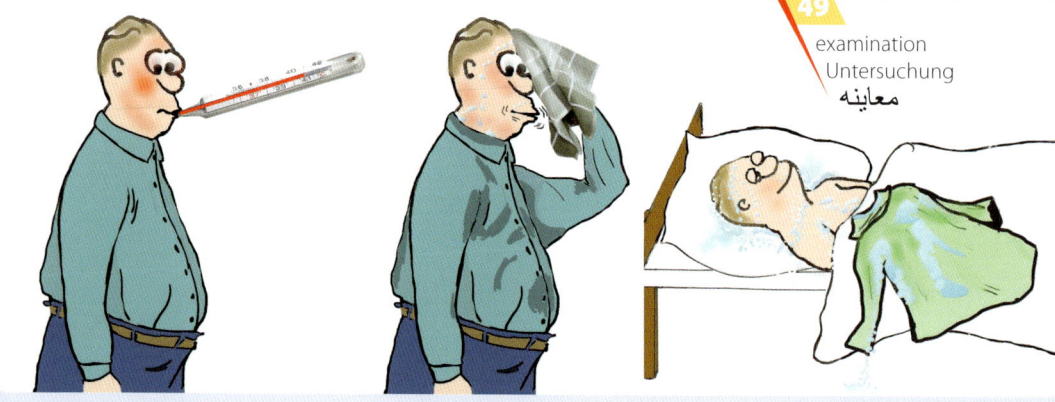

49 examination / Untersuchung / معاینه

fever	sweating	night sweats
Fieber	schwitzen	Nachtschweiß
تب	عرق ریختن	عرق وقت خواب

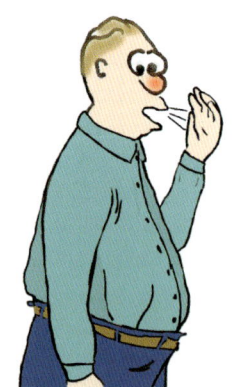 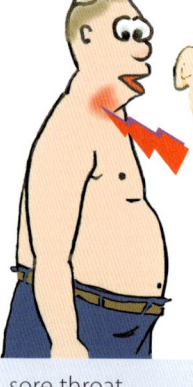 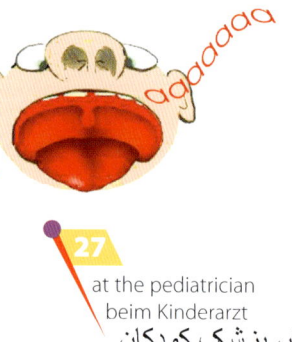

27 at the pediatrician / beim Kinderarzt / پیش پزشک کودکان

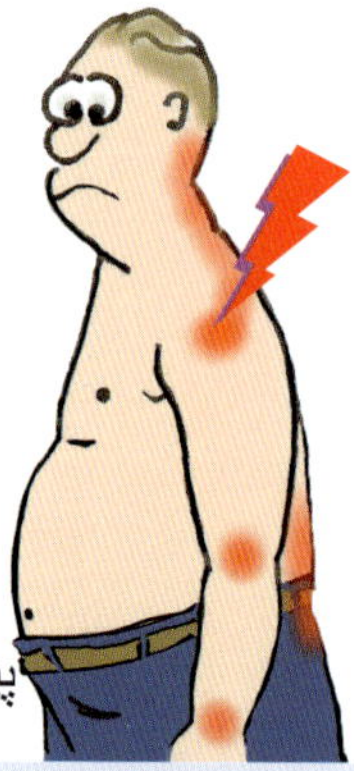

coughing	cold	sore throat	cold	pain in the limbs
Husten	Schnupfen	Halsschmerzen	Erkältung	Gliederschmerzen
سرفه	آبریزش بینی	گلودرد	سرماخوردگی	کوفتگی

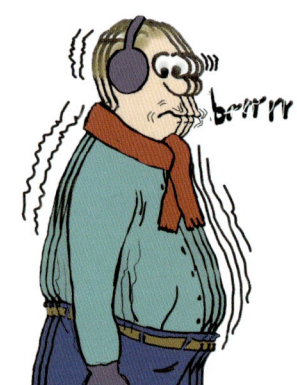 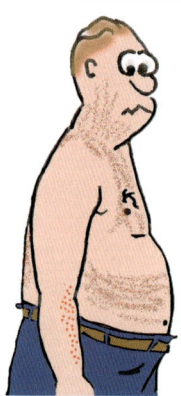 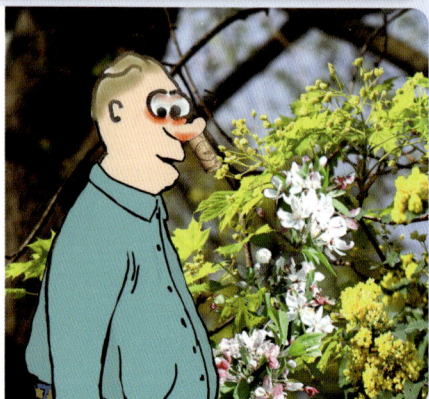

shivering	allergy	hay-fever
Frösteln	Allergie	Heuschnupfen
لرز	حساسیت	سرماخوردگی بهاری

At the family doctor
Pain/sensitivity

Beim Hausarzt
Schmerzen/Missempfindungen

پیش پزشک خانواده
دردها / احساسهای بد

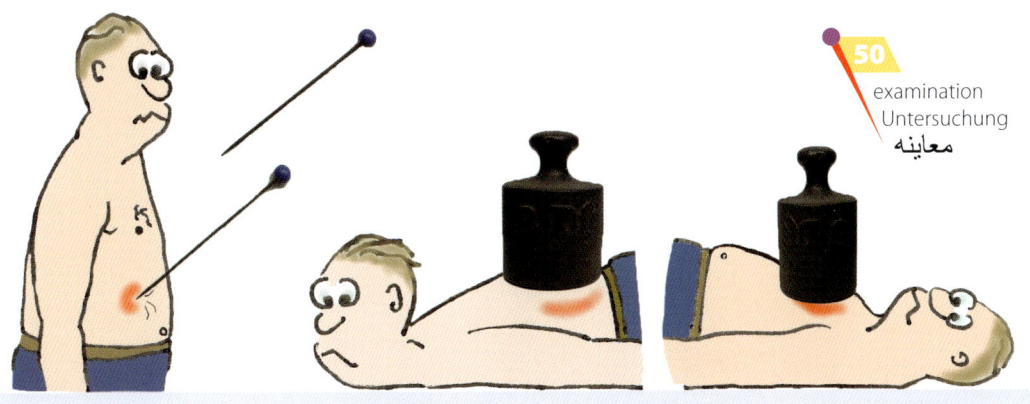

50
examination
Untersuchung
معاینه

piercing pain
spitzer Schmerz
درد نقطه ای

dull or blunt pain
dumpfer oder stumpfer Schmerz
درد خفیف یا نامعلوم

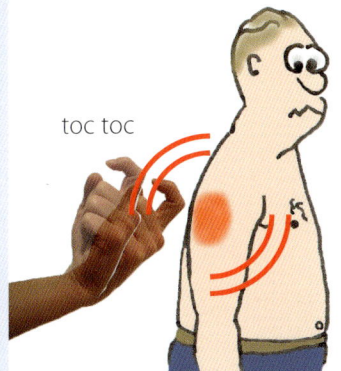

toc toc

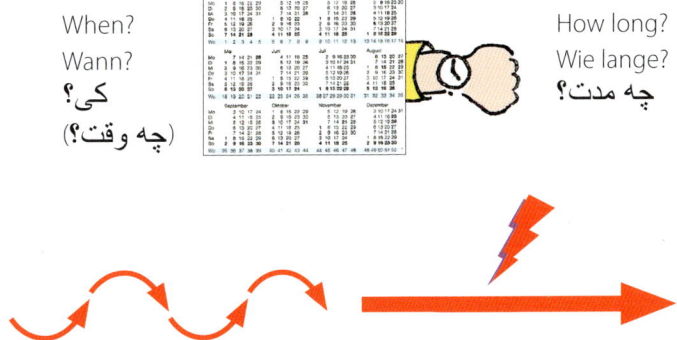

When?
Wann?
کی؟
(چه وقت؟)

How long?
Wie lange?
چه مدت؟

throbbing
klopfend
ضربه ای

wave-like/convulsive
wellenförmig/krampfartig
موجی شکل / گرفتگی

always the same
immer gleich
پیوسته

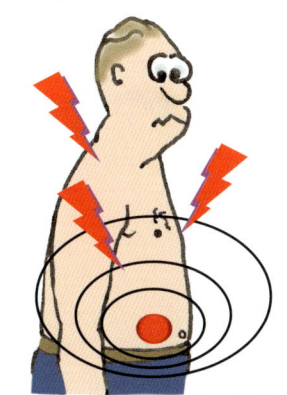

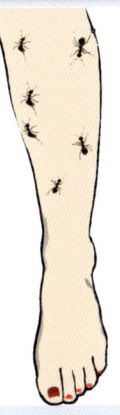

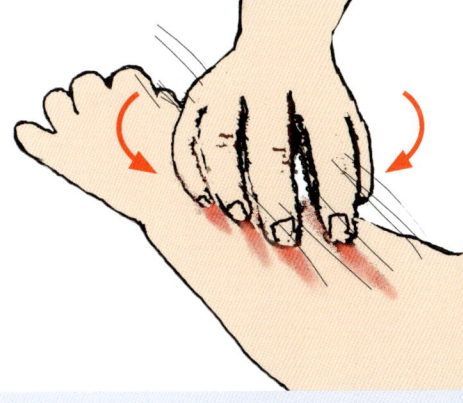

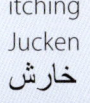

radiation
Ausstrahlung
تشعشع

tickling/needles and pins
Kribbeln/Ameisen
وول زدن زیر پوست / مورچه

itching
Jucken
خارش

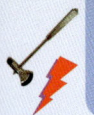

At the family doctor
Pain/nerves

Beim Hausarzt
Schmerzen/Nerven

پیش پزشک خانواده
دردها / اعصاب

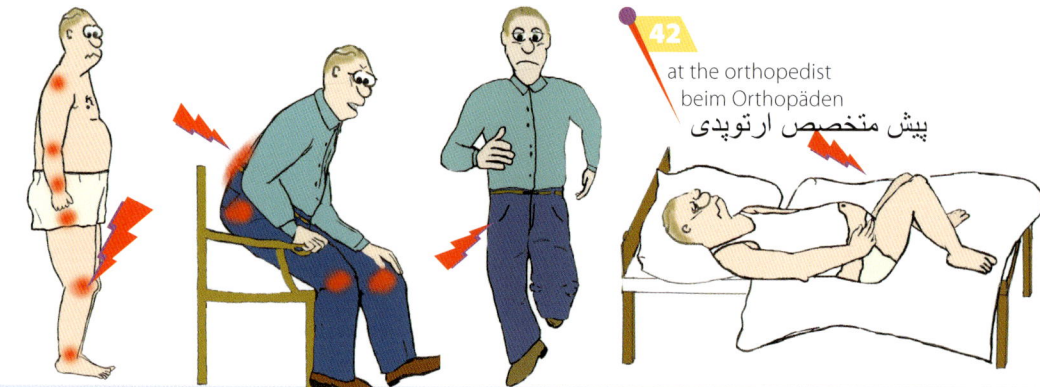

42 at the orthopedist
beim Orthopäden
پیش متخصص ارتوپدی

pain in the joints	start-up pain	while moving	when resting
Gelenkschmerzen	Anlaufschmerz	bei Bewegung	in Ruhe
درد مفصلی	درد وقت دورخیز	در حرکت	وقت استراحت

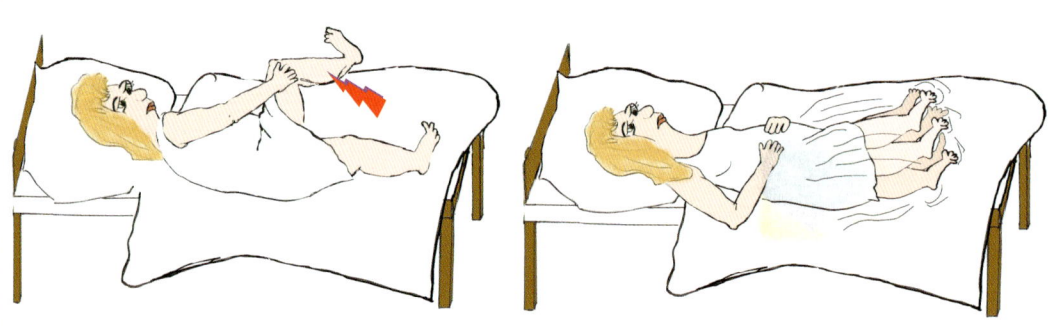

cramps in the legs
Krämpfe in den Beinen/Wadenkrämpfe
گرفتگی عضلات پا

twitching in the legs at night
nachts Zuckungen in den Beinen
لرز در پاها وقت خواب

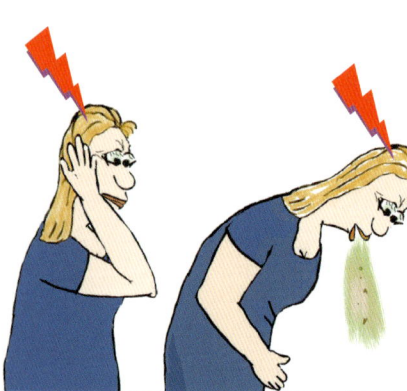
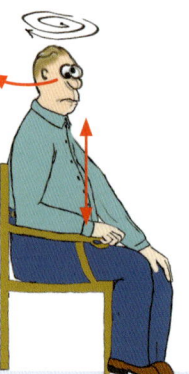
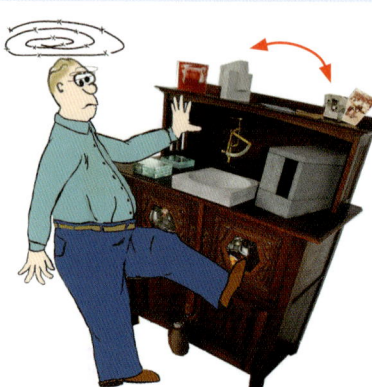

headache	with vomiting	like a merry-go-round	I´m tumbling.
Kopfschmerzen	mit Erbrechen	Es dreht sich alles.	Ich taumele, schwanke.
سردرد	با حالت تهوع	سرگیجه دارم.	من تلو تلو میخورم.

At the family doctor
Nerves

Beim Hausarzt
Nerven

پیش پزشک خانواده
اعصاب

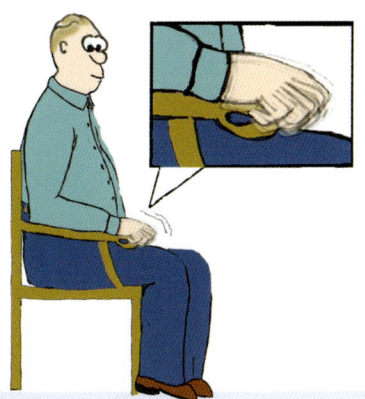
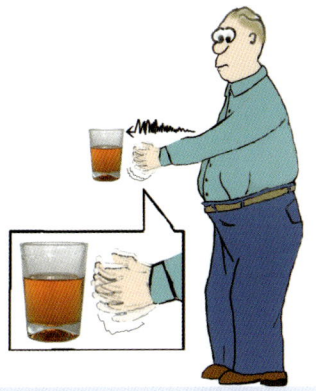
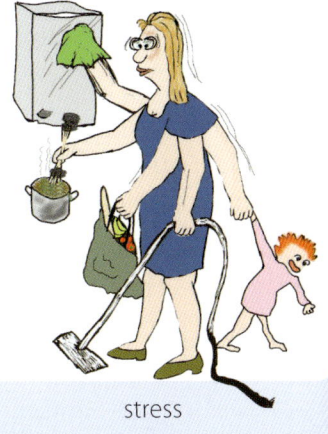

tremble while resting
Zittern in Ruhe
لرزش دائمی

tremble when moving
Zittern bei Bewegung
لرزش در حرکت

stress
Stress
استرس

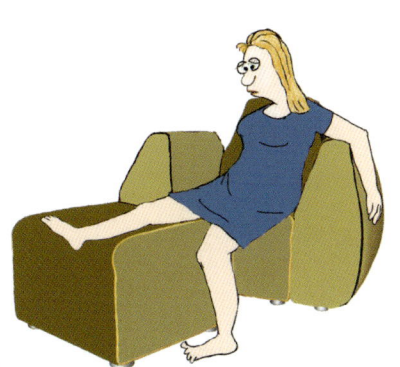
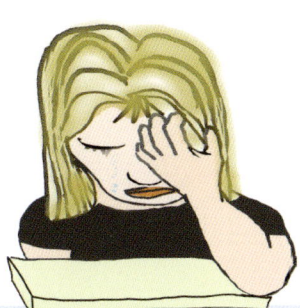
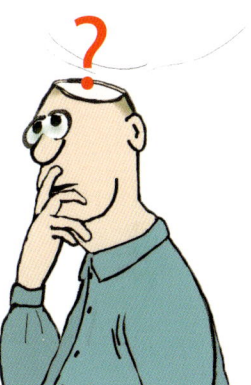

exhaustion
Abgeschlagenheit
خستگی

depression
Depression
افسردگی

forgetfulness
Vergesslichkeit
فراموشکاری

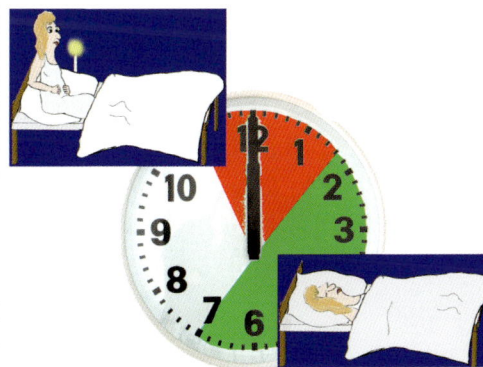
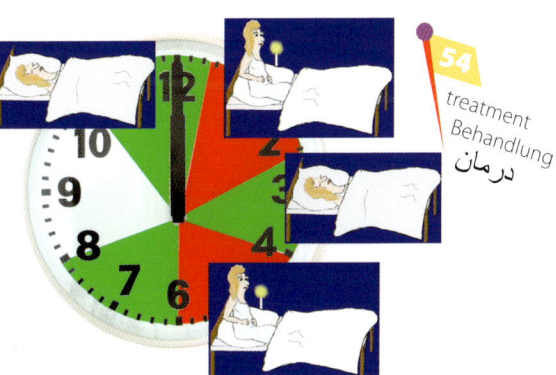

treatment
Behandlung
درمان

troubles falling asleep
Einschlafstörung
اختلالات وقت خوابیدن

troubles sleeping through the night
Durchschlafstörung
بدخوابی

At the family doctor / Beim Hausarzt
Heart/circulation — Herz/Kreislauf

پیش پزشک خانواده
قلب / گردش خون

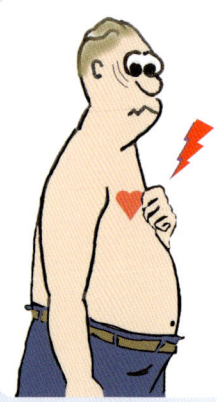
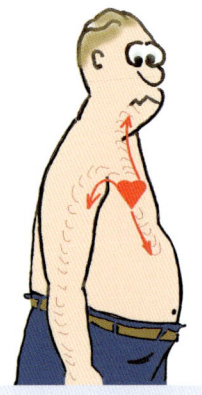
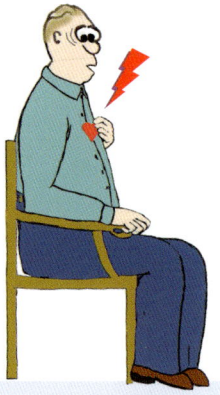
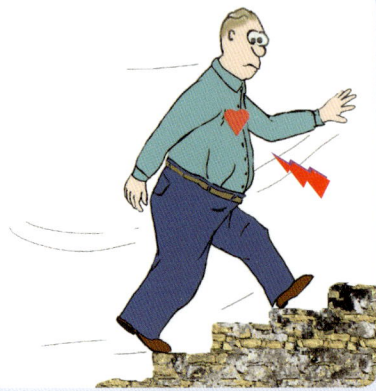

heartache	radiation	while resting	during physical exertion
Herzschmerzen	Ausstrahlung	in Ruhe	bei Anstrengung
درد ناحیه قلبی	تشعشع	هنگام نشستن	وقت تلاش وتقلا

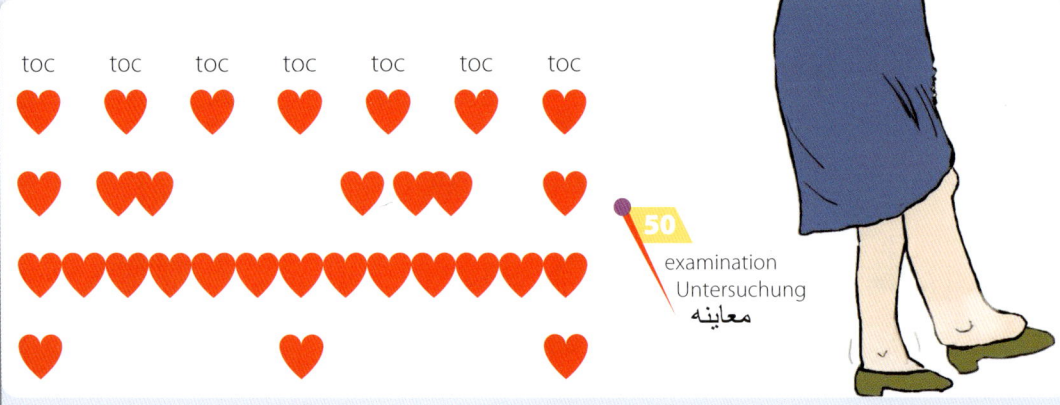

examination
Untersuchung
معاینه

palpitations/heart rhythm	swollen ankles in the evening
Herzstolpern/Herzrhythmus	abends dicke Knöchel
طپش قلب / ضربان قلب	قوزک متورم پا بعد از کار روزانه

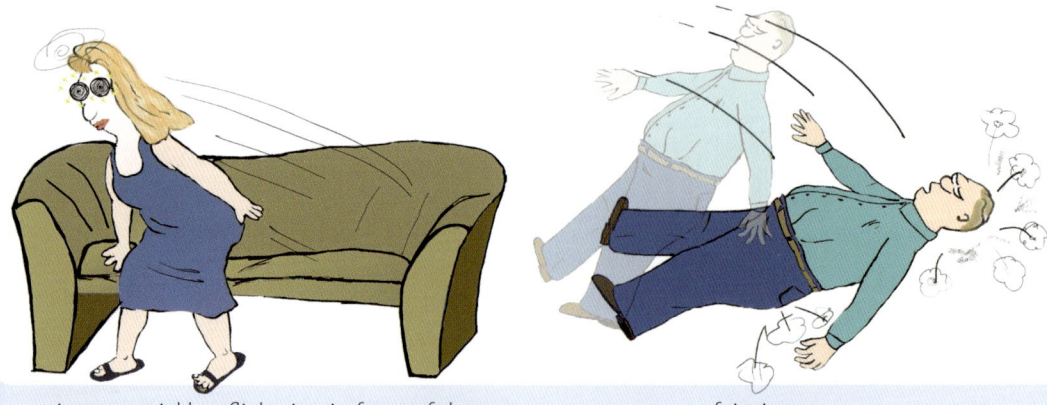

getting up quickly – flickering in front of the eyes	fainting
schnell aufstehen – Flimmern vor Augen	Ohnmacht
بلند شدن سریع - سیاهی رفتن چشمها	بیهوشی

At the family doctor
Circulation/breathing

Beim Hausarzt
Kreislauf/Atmung

پیش پزشک خانواده
گردش خون / تنفس

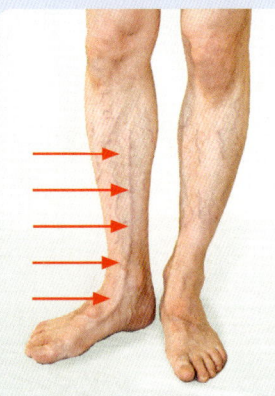
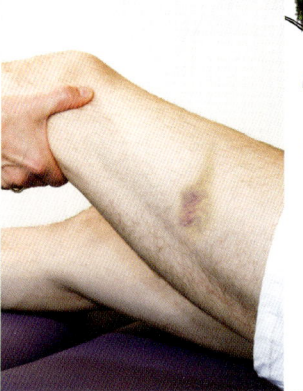
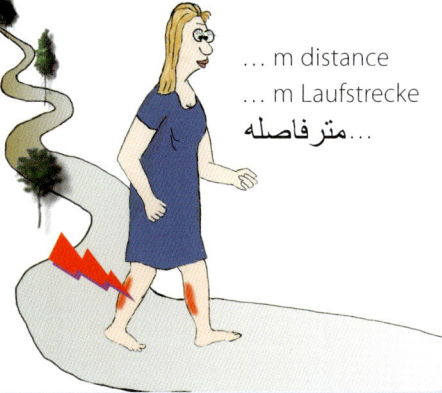

... m distance
... m Laufstrecke
...متر فاصله

varicose veins
Krampfadern
واریس

disposition to bruises
leicht blaue Flecken
گرایش به کبودی پوست

pain in the legs
Schmerzen in den Beinen
پا درد

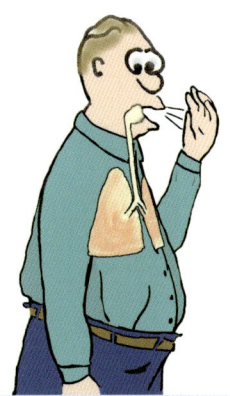
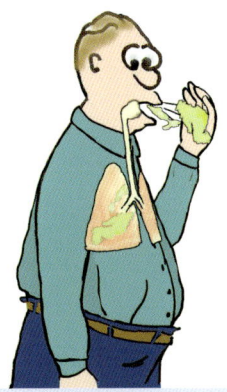
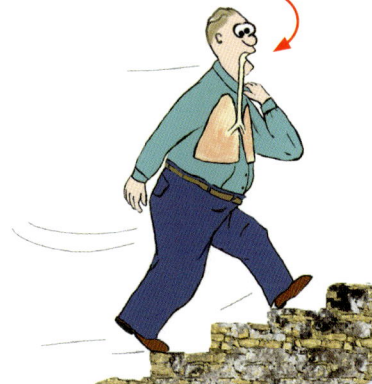

dry cough
trockener Husten
سرفه خشک

with phlegm
mit Auswurf
با خلط

shortness of breath during exertion
Luftnot bei Anstrengung
نفس تنگی وقت تلاش و تقلا

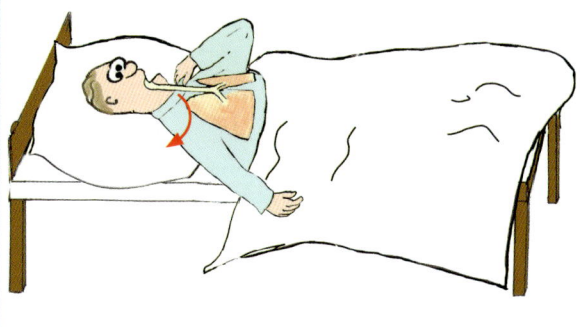
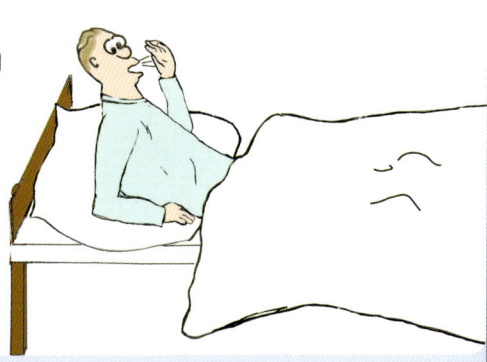

suffocation attack/at night
Erstickungsanfälle/nachts
احساس خفگی / شبها

nocturnal cough
nächtlicher Husten
سرفه طبیعی

At the family doctor
Stomach

Beim Hausarzt
Magen

پیش پزشک خانواده
معده

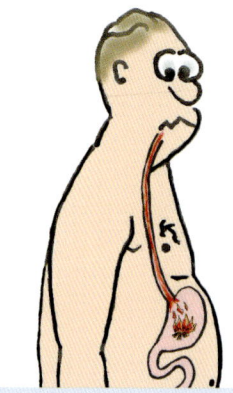
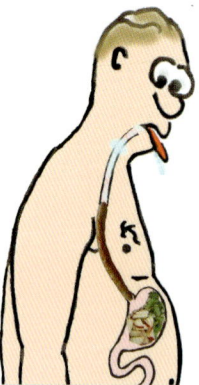
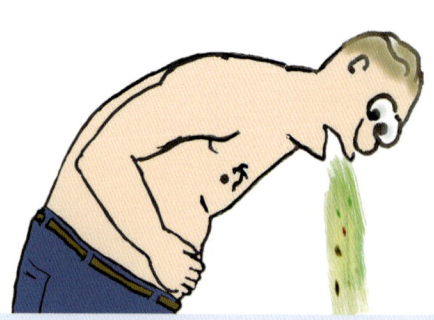

heartburn	nausea	vomiting
Sodbrennen	Übelkeit	Erbrechen
سوزش معده	حالت تهوع	استفراغ

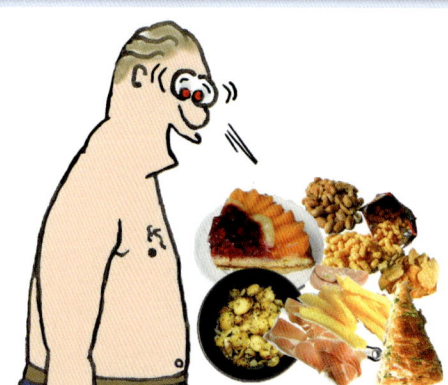
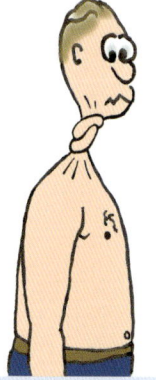
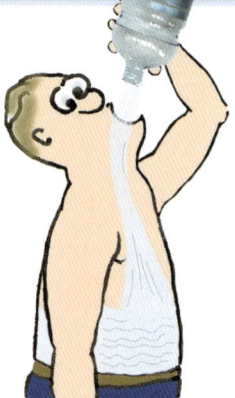

extreme (abnormal) appetite	lack of appetite	thirstiness
Heißhunger	Appetitlosigkeit	Durstgefühl
اشتهای ناگهانی	بی اشتهائی	تشنگی

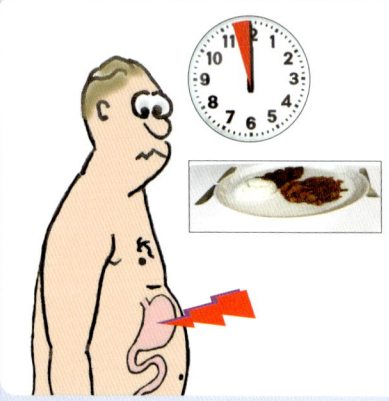
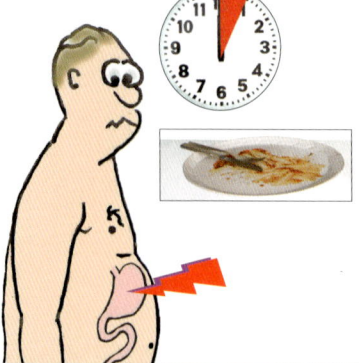
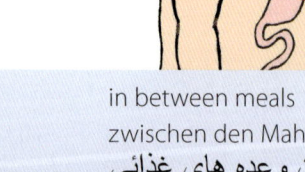

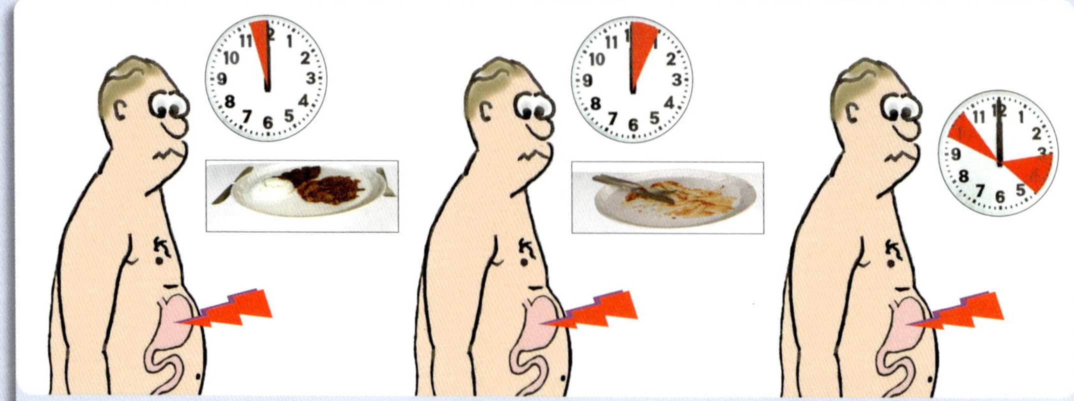

stomachache	before	after	in between meals
Magenschmerzen	vor	nach	zwischen den Mahlzeiten
معده درد	قبل	بعد	بین وعده های غذائی

At the family doctor
Bowles

Beim Hausarzt
Darm

پیش پزشک خانواده
روده

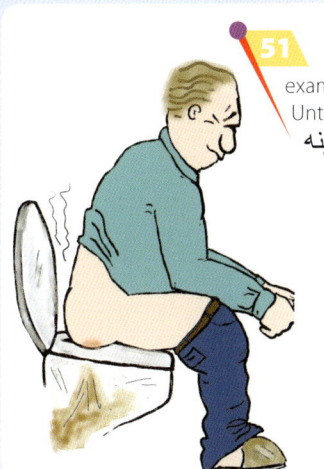

51 examination / Untersuchung / معاینه

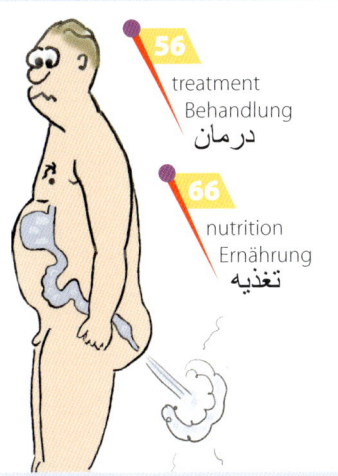

56 treatment / Behandlung / درمان

66 nutrition / Ernährung / تغذیه

diarrhoea
Durchfall
اسهال

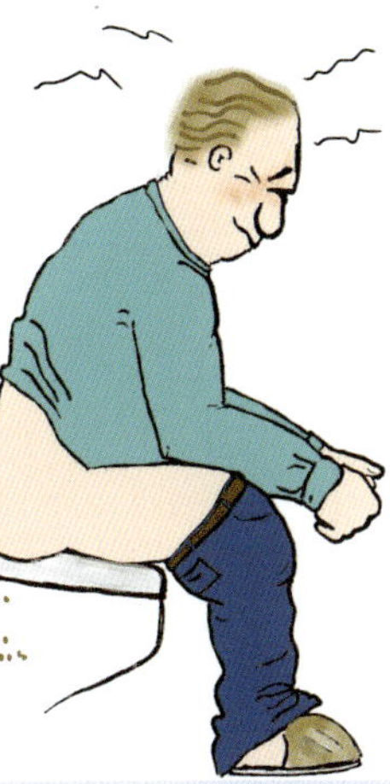

constipation
Verstopfung
یبوست

gas
Blähungen
نفخ

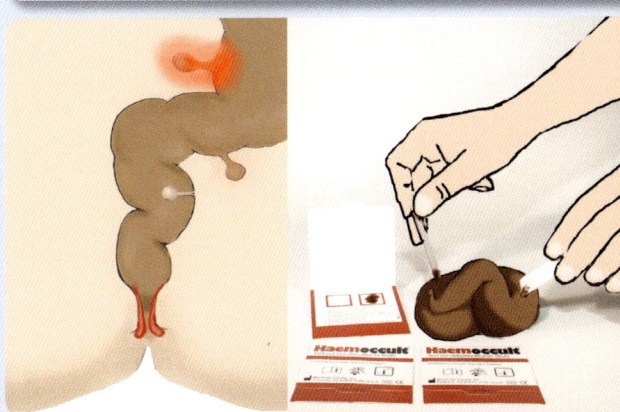

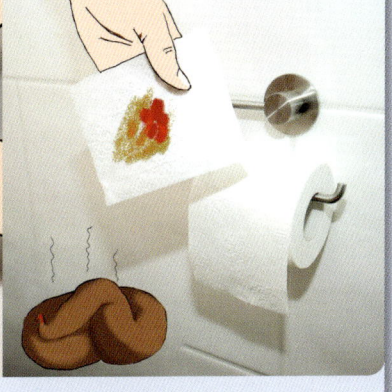

diverticula, polyp, haemorrhoids
Divertikel, Polyp, Hämorrhoiden
بواسیر، عفونت روده ، پولیپ روده

bowel cancer prevention
Darmkrebsvorsorge
پیشگیری سرطان روده

blood when wiping
Blut beim Abputzen
خون در وقت تمیزکردن مقعد

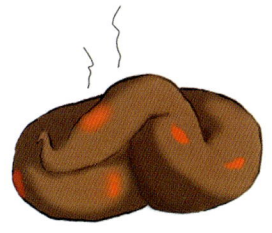

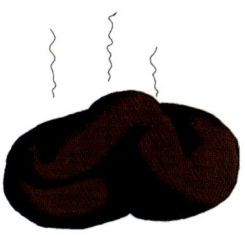

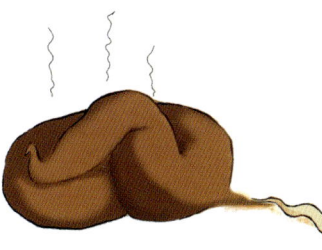

blood on the stool
Blutauflagerungen
مدفوع خونی

black stool
schwarzer Stuhlgang
مدفوع سیاه رنگ

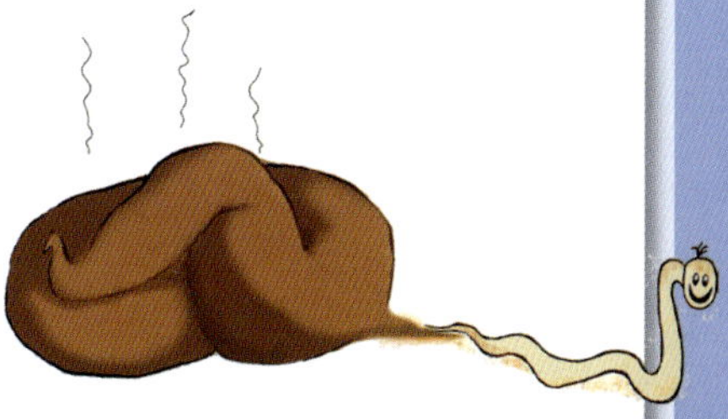

worms
Würmer
کرمها

19

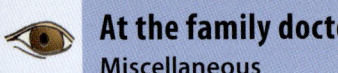

At the family doctor — **Beim Hausarzt** — پیش پزشک خانواده
Miscellaneous — Sonstiges — موارد دیگر

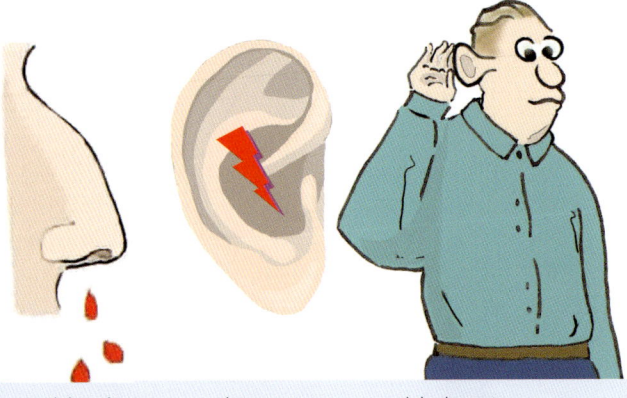

nose-bleeding	earache	trouble hearing	ringing in the ears
Nasenbluten	Ohrenschmerzen	Schwerhörigkeit	Ohrgeräusch
خون دماغ	گوش درد	کم شنوائی	سروصدا در گوش

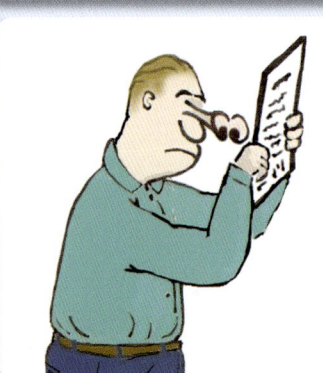 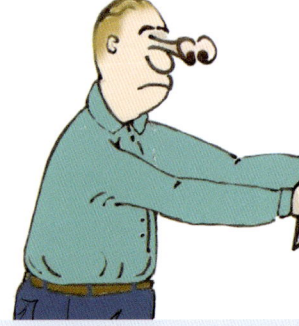 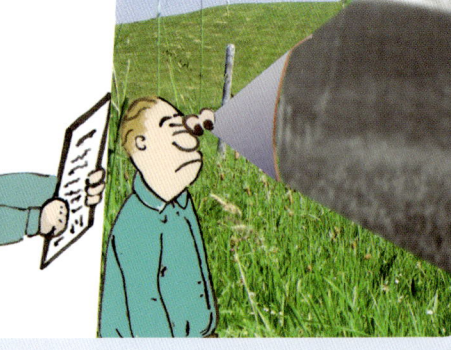

short-sighted	long-sighted	cloudy vision
kurzsichtig	weitsichtig	Grauschleier / grauer Star
نزدیک بین	دوربین	آب مروارید

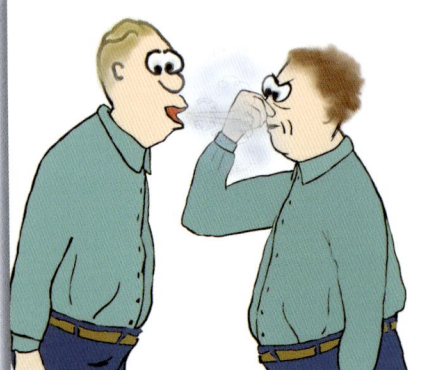 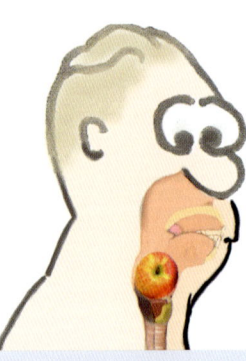 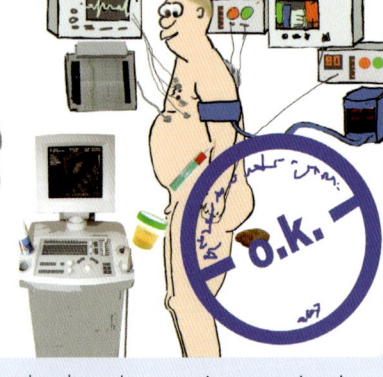

bad breath	difficulties swallowing	only check-up/preventive examination
Mundgeruch	Schluckbeschwerden	nur Kontrolle/ Vorsorge
بوی بد دهان	مشکل هنگام قورت دادن	فقط کنترل / پیشگیری

STUTTGART

Landeshauptstadt Stuttgart
Abteilung für Integrationspolitik

Die Abteilung für Integrations-politik hat den Auftrag, die Umsetzung der Stuttgarter integrationspolitischen Ziele zu initiieren, zu moderieren und zu koordinieren.

Die Ziele sind:
1. Die Förderung der gesellschaftlichen Partizipation und der Chancengleichheit von Menschen unterschiedlicher Herkunft.
2. Die Förderung des friedlichen Zusammenlebens der verschiedenen Bevölkerungsgruppen.
3. Die Nutzung der kulturellen Vielfalt als Potenzial für die internationale Stadtgemeinschaft.

Das Stuttgarter Bündnis für Integration
Das Integrationskonzept „Stuttgarter Bündnis für Integration" wird als eine gemeinsame Aufgabe von allen beteiligten gesellschaftlichen Gruppen mitgetragen und umgesetzt.

Zu den Bündnispartnern zählen, neben den zahlreichen Institutionen, Bürgerinnen und Bürger mit und ohne deutschen Pass sowie ihre Vereine. Auch 30 interkulturelle Gesundheitsmediatoren des Projekts MiMi gehören dazu. Das Projekt wird am Standort Stuttgart von der Abteilung für Integrationspolitik koordiniert.

Weitere Informationen dazu unter www.stuttgart.de/Integrationspolitik.

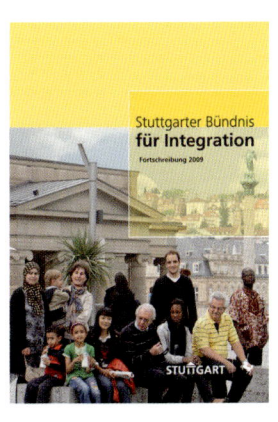

VIA e.V. ist ein Dachverband für Vereine, Gruppen und Initiativen, die in der Migranten-, Aussiedler- und Flüchtlingsarbeit aktiv sind.

Bundesweit sind über 100 Organisationen im Verband organisiert. Hinzu kommen weitere Einrichtungen aus dem europäischen Ausland.
Ein wichtiger Arbeitsschwerpunkt für VIA ist "Migration und Gesundheit". Im Projekt **"Gesundheit für Migranten/innen - Sensibilisierung und Prävention"** geht es neben Informationsvermittlung über das deutsche Gesundheitssystem vor allem um den Aufbau von gesundheitlichen Präventionskursen für Migrantinnen und Migranten.

Näheres auf der VIA-Homepage:
www.via-bundesverband.de

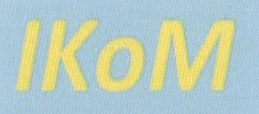

Informations- und Kontaktstelle für die Arbeit mit älteren MigrantInnen

Das bietet Ihnen IKoM:

✓ Umfangreichen Fachnewsletter
✓ Literatur- und Kontaktdatenbank
✓ Informationen zu Projekten, Veranstaltungen und Neuerscheinungen
✓ Vernetzung

Kontakt:
Aktion Courage e.V.
Kaiserstr. 201
53113 Bonn
Tel.: 0228-92129358
E-Mail: ikom@aktioncourage.org
Homepage: www.ikom-bund.de

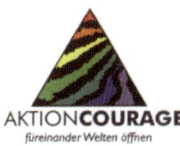

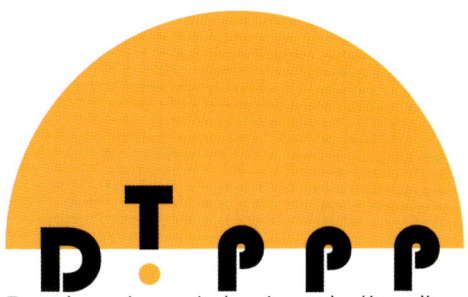

Dachverband der transkulturellen Psychiatrie, Psychotherapie und Psychosomatik im deutschsprachigen Raum e.V.

Postfach 26 22 • D-59016 Hamm •
www.dtppp.com • info@dtppp.com

G O U R M A N D
world cookbook awards **2004**

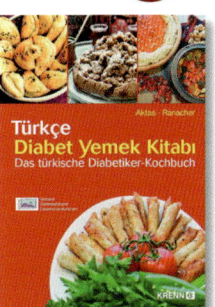

Das türkische Diabetiker-Kochbuch

Kitabımızda yaşam kalitesine uygun geleneksel türk mutfağına özgu yemek tariflerini bulacaksınız.
Diabet üzerine, Yüksek şeker belirtileri.
ABC Diabet.

ISBN 978-3-902351-27-2   www.hubertkrenn.at

| Organs | Organe | اعضای بدن |

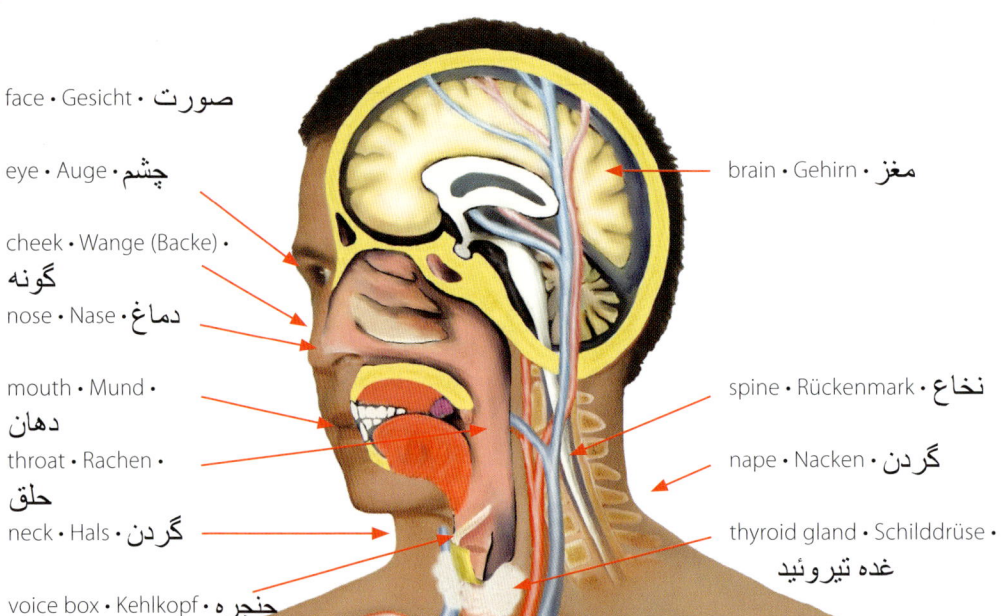

face • Gesicht • صورت
eye • Auge • چشم
cheek • Wange (Backe) • گونه
nose • Nase • دماغ
mouth • Mund • دهان
throat • Rachen • حلق
neck • Hals • گردن
voice box • Kehlkopf • حنجره

brain • Gehirn • مغز
spine • Rückenmark • نخاع
nape • Nacken • گردن
thyroid gland • Schilddrüse • غده تیروئید

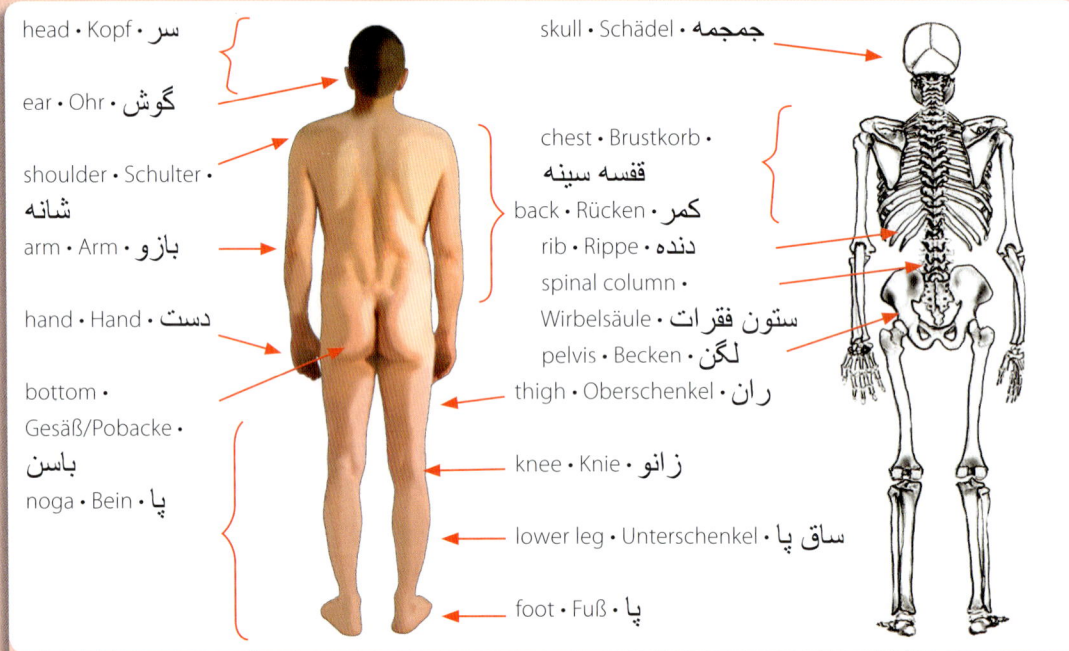

head • Kopf • سر
ear • Ohr • گوش
shoulder • Schulter • شانه
arm • Arm • بازو
hand • Hand • دست
bottom • Gesäß/Pobacke • باسن
noga • Bein • پا

skull • Schädel • جمجمه
chest • Brustkorb • قفسه سینه
back • Rücken • کمر
rib • Rippe • دنده
spinal column • Wirbelsäule • ستون فقرات
pelvis • Becken • لگن
thigh • Oberschenkel • ران
knee • Knie • زانو
lower leg • Unterschenkel • ساق پا
foot • Fuß • پا

My problems are here – point to e. g. an area or an organ
Ich habe dort Probleme – zeigen Sie z. B. auf ein Gebiet oder Organ
اینجا مشکل دارم.

Organs • Organe • اعضای بدن

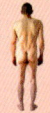

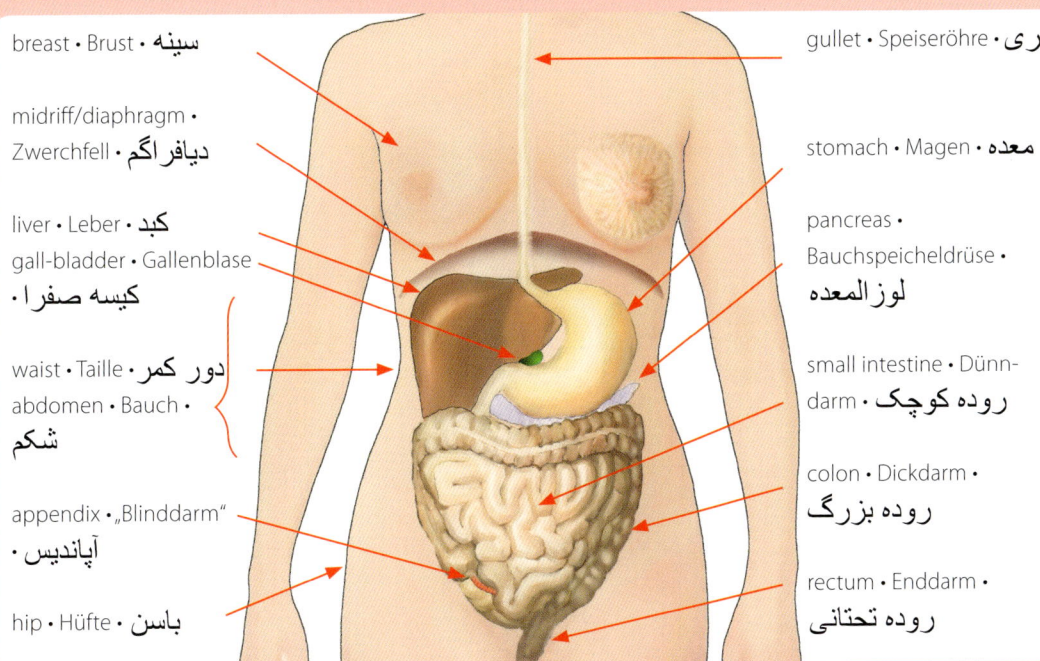

- breast • Brust • سینه
- midriff/diaphragm • Zwerchfell • دیافراگم
- liver • Leber • کبد
- gall-bladder • Gallenblase • کیسه صفرا
- waist • Taille • دور کمر
- abdomen • Bauch • شکم
- appendix • „Blinddarm" • آپاندیس
- hip • Hüfte • باسن
- gullet • Speiseröhre • مری
- stomach • Magen • معده
- pancreas • Bauchspeicheldrüse • لوزالمعده
- small intestine • Dünndarm • روده کوچک
- colon • Dickdarm • روده بزرگ
- rectum • Enddarm • روده تحتانی

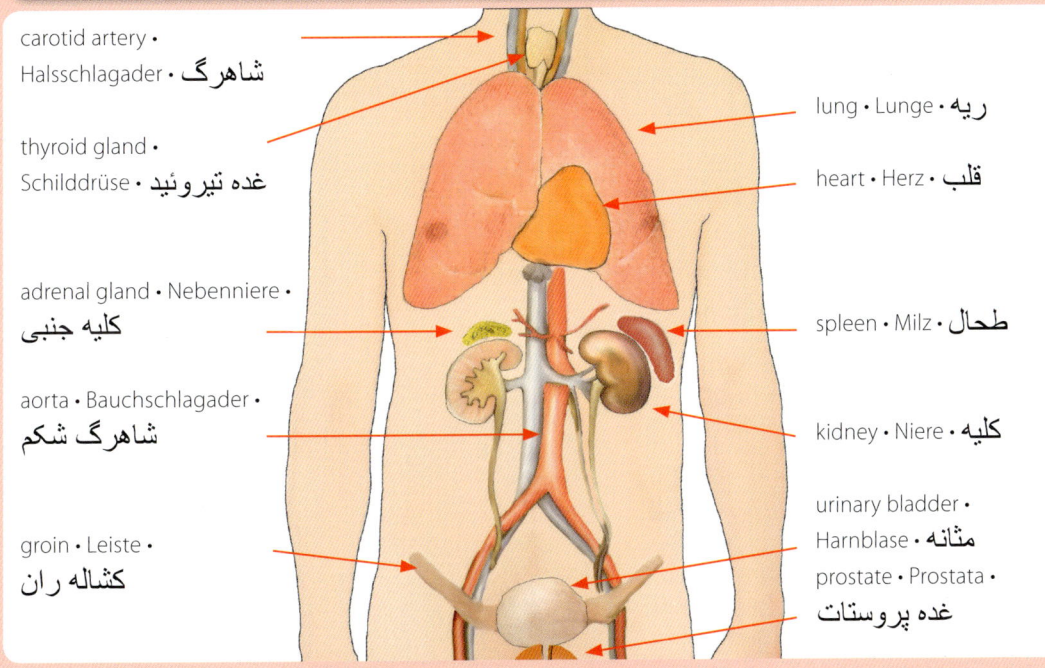

- carotid artery • Halsschlagader • شاهرگ
- thyroid gland • Schilddrüse • غده تیروئید
- adrenal gland • Nebenniere • کلیه جنبی
- aorta • Bauchschlagader • شاهرگ شکم
- groin • Leiste • کشاله ران
- lung • Lunge • ریه
- heart • Herz • قلب
- spleen • Milz • طحال
- kidney • Niere • کلیه
- urinary bladder • Harnblase • مثانه
- prostate • Prostata • غده پروستات

My problems are here – point to e. g. an area or an organ
Ich habe dort Probleme – zeigen Sie z. B. auf ein Gebiet oder Organ
اینجا مشکل دارم.

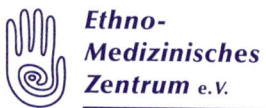

Ethno-Medizinisches Zentrum e.V.

www.ethno-medizinisches-zentrum.de

Das MiMi-Projekt:
"Mit Migranten für Migranten – Interkulturelle Gesundheit in Deutschland"

Migrantinnen und Migranten sind angesichts spezifischer Hindernisse, wie etwa Fremdsprachigkeit oder der fehlenden Vertrautheit mit den Verhältnissen im deutschen Gesundheitssystem, beim Zugang zu Informationen, Beratung und Therapien oftmals benachteiligt. Um einer Fehl- oder Unterversorgung entgegenzuwirken, wurde 2003 das Projekt „MiMi – Mit Migranten für Migranten – Interkulturelle Gesundheit in Deutschland" vom Ethno-Medizinischen Zentrum e.V. (EMZ) entwickelt. Ziel des Projekts ist es, mehrsprachige und kultursensible Gesundheitsförderung und Prävention für Migrantinnen und Migranten anzubieten.

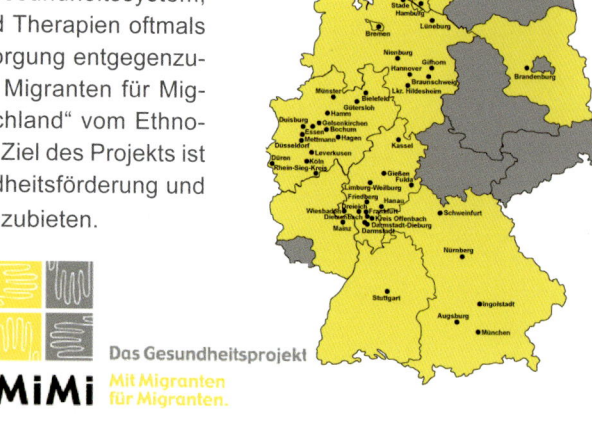

Dazu werden engagierte Menschen mit Migrationshintergrund zu interkulturellen Gesundheitsmediatoren ausgebildet, die dann als Multiplikatoren ihre Landsleute in der jeweiligen Muttersprache zum deutschen Gesundheitssystem und weiteren Themen der Gesundheitsförderung und Prävention informieren. Gegenwärtig wird das MiMi-Gesundheitsprojekt an mehr als 50 Orten und in 10 Bundesländern durchgeführt. Schirmherrin des Projekts ist die Bundesbeauftragte für Migration, Integration und Flüchtlinge, Staatsministerin Prof. Dr. Maria Böhmer.

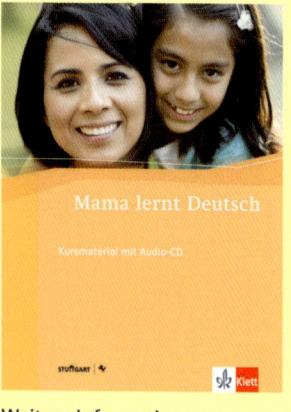

Mama lernt Deutsch
Kursmaterial mit Audio-CD
978-3-12-676190-1

- Deutsch für das tägliche Leben
- mit den Themen Schule, Familie, Gesundheit

Weitere Informationen:
www.klett.de/MamalerntDeutsch

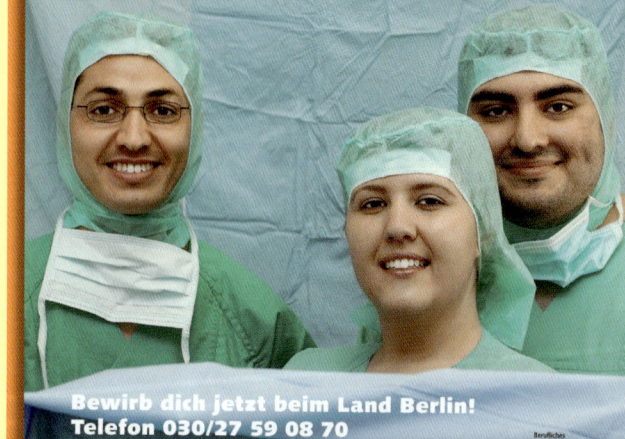

Berlin braucht dich!

Berlin potrzebuje ciebie!
Берлин нуждается в тебе!
Berlin needs you!
Berlin'in sana ihtiyacı var!
Berlin cân ban!
برلين بحاجة اليك!

Bewirb dich jetzt beim Land Berlin!
Telefon 030/27 59 08 70
www.berlin-braucht-dich.de

BQNBerlin

At the pediatrician
Questions

Beim Kinderarzt
Fragen

پیش پزشک کودکان
سوالها

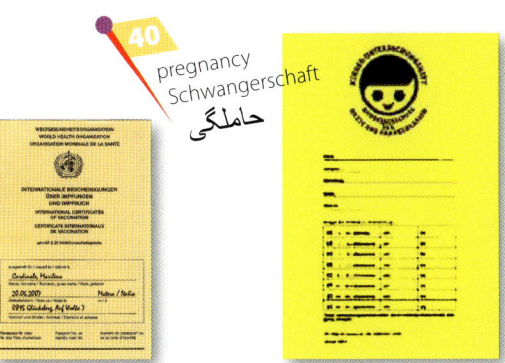

pregnancy
Schwangerschaft
حاملگی

Certificate of Vaccination | Prevention Card | Maternity Card
Impfpass | Vorsorgeheft | Mutterpass
دفترچه واکسن | دفترچه پیشگیری | دفترچه حاملگی

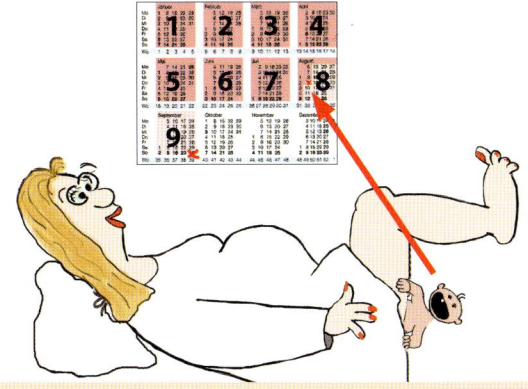
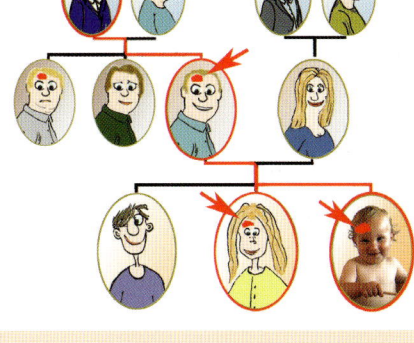

preterm delivery
Frühgeburt
زایمان زودرس

family diseases
Familienkrankheiten
بیماریهای ارثی

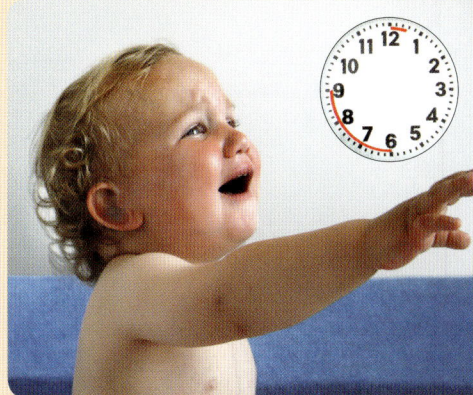
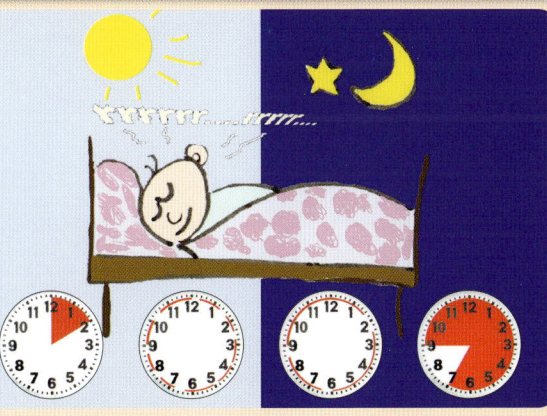

screaming
Schreien
گریه کردن نوزاد

midday nap – sleeping-rhythm – sleeping through the night
Mittagsschlaf – Schlafrhythmus – Durchschlafen
خواب ظهر - ریتم خواب - خواب طولانی

25

At the pediatrician
Nutrition

Beim Kinderarzt
Ernährung

پیش پزشک کودکان
تغذیه

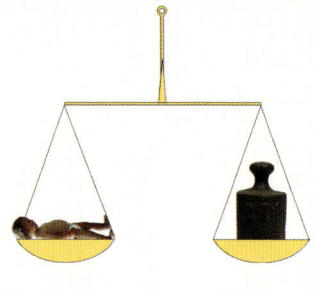
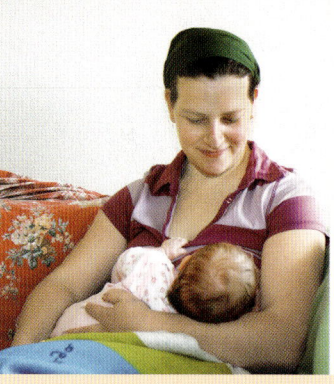
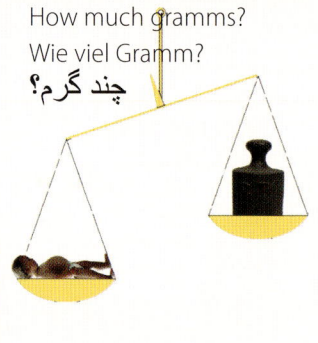

weigh before
vorher wiegen
قبل از شیر دادن وزن کنید.

breast feeding
stillen
شیر بدهید.

weigh afterward
nachher wiegen
بعد از شیر دادن وزن کنید.

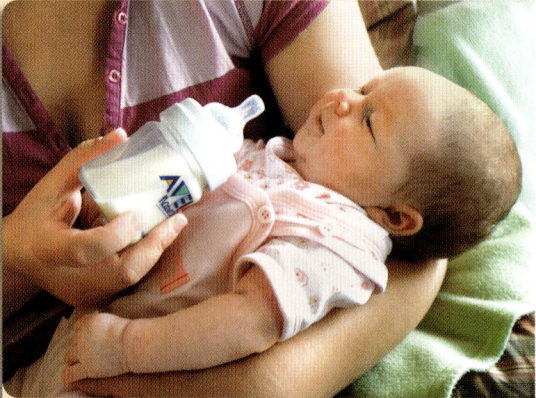
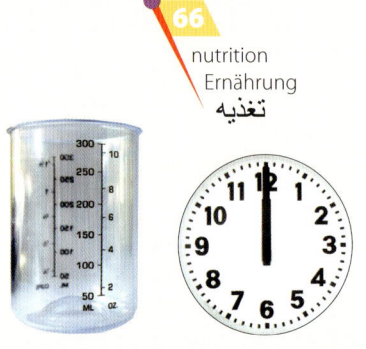

nutrition
Ernährung
تغذیه

milk bottle
Milchflasche
شیشه شیر

How much ml is the child drinking? How often?
Wie viel ml trinkt das Kind? Wie oft?
نوزاد شما چند سی سی شیر میخورد؟ چند بار؟

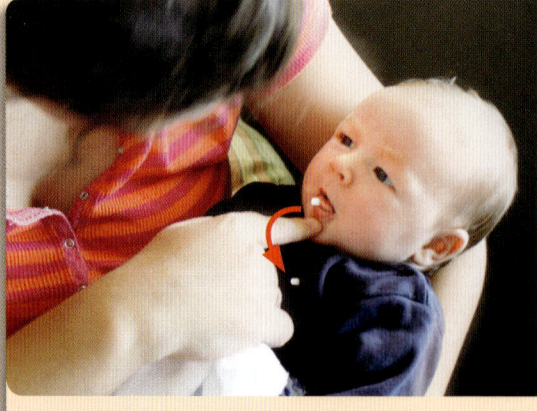
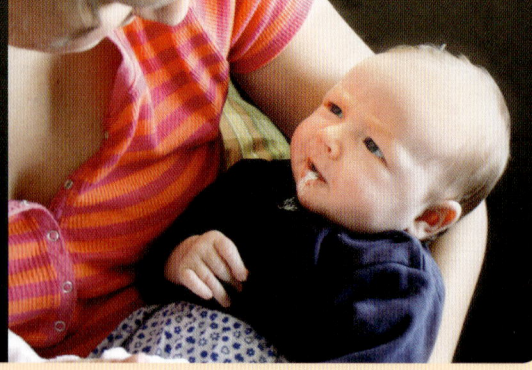

spitting the medicine
Medikament ausgespuckt
تف کردن دارو

spew
Spucken/Speien
استفراغ کردن / بالا آوردن

At the pediatrician
Troubles/inoculation

Beim Kinderarzt
Beschwerden/Impfung

پیش پزشک کودکان
ناراحتیها / واکسیناسیون

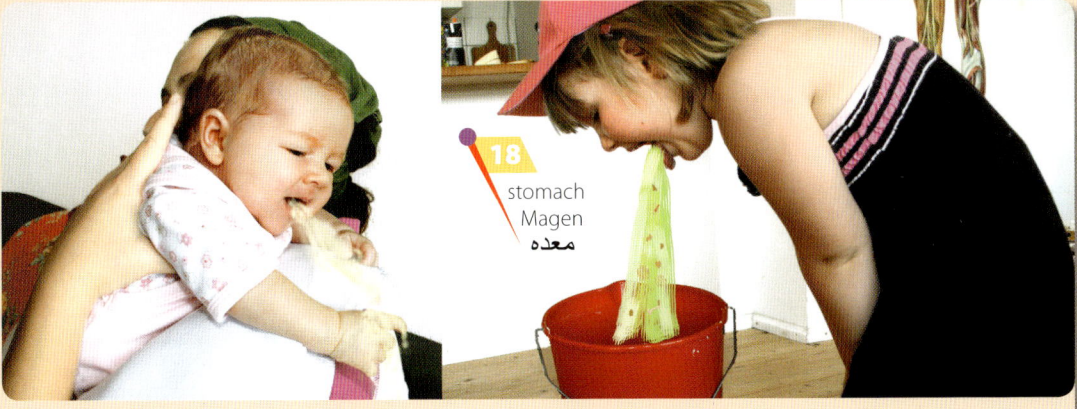

18 stomach / Magen / معده

torential vomiting
Erbrechen im Schwall
استفراغ مداوم

sickness
Erbrechen
استفراغ

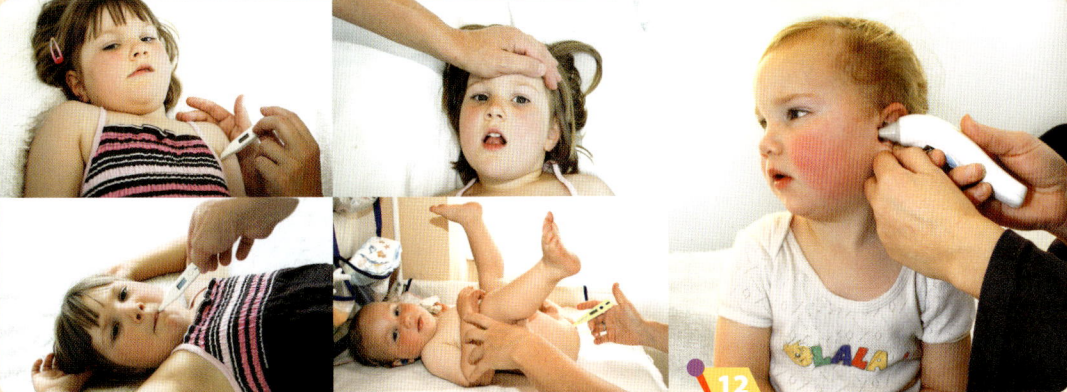

12 cold
Erkältung, Schnupfen
آبریزش بینی، سرماخوردگی

taking the temperature – where and how taken?
Fieber messen – wo und wie gemessen?
اندازه گیری تب – کجا و چگونه اندازه گیری شده؟

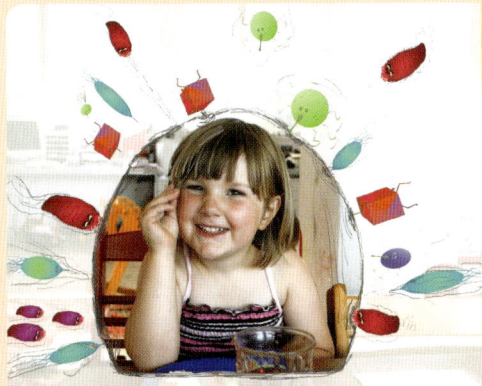
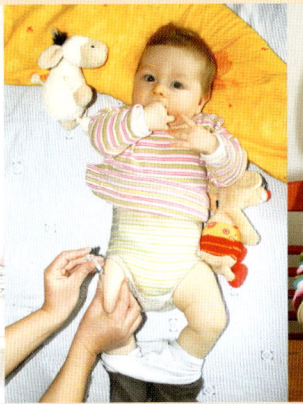
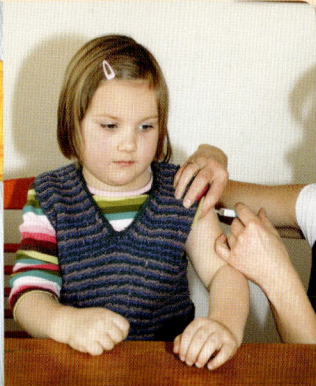

inoculation
Impfung
واکسیناسیون

basic immunisation
Grundimmunisierung
واکسیناسیون پایه

refresh
Auffrischung
یاد آوری

At the pediatrician
Troubles

Beim Kinderarzt
Beschwerden

پیش پزشک کودکان
ناراحتیها

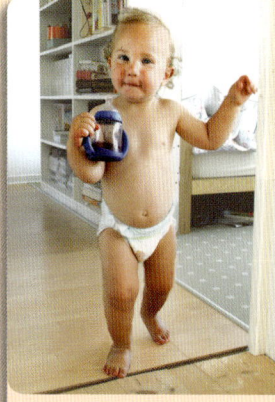 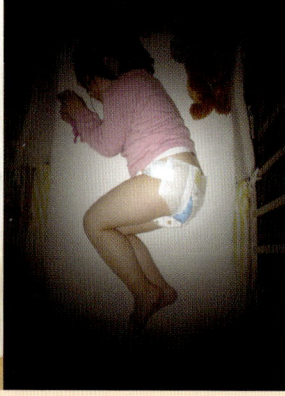 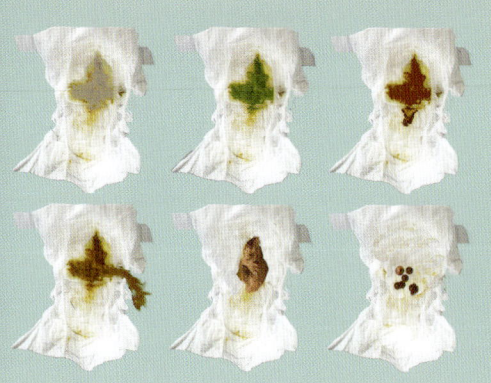

diapers during the night/day
Windeln nachts/tags
پوشک کردن شبها / روزها

digestion
Verdauung
هضم غذا

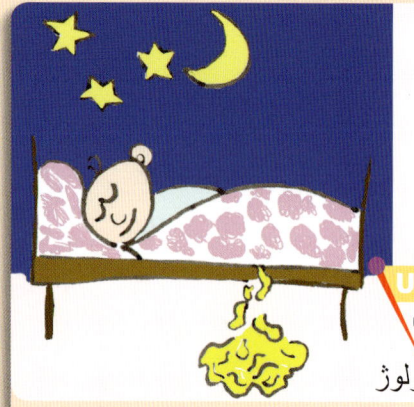 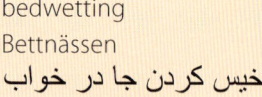 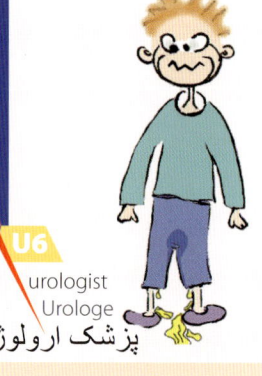 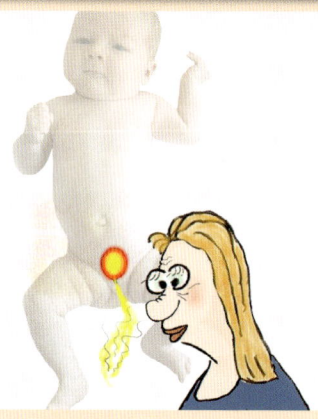

urologist
Urologe
پزشک ارولوژ

bedwetting
Bettnässen
خیس کردن جا در خواب

wetting by day
Einnässen bei Tag
خیس کردن جا در روز

urine smells strong
Urin riecht
ادرار بوی بد میدهد.

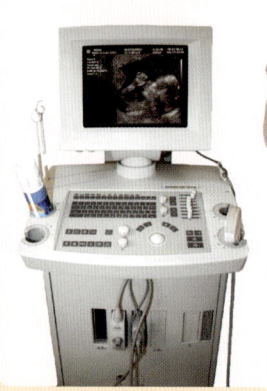 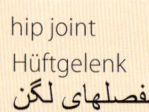 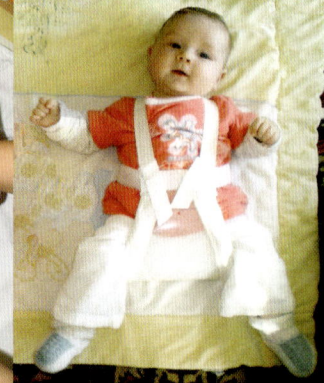

routine check
Routinekontrolle
کنترل روتین

hip joint
Hüftgelenk
مفصلهای لگن

hip dysplasia
Hüftgelenksdysplasie
نقص عضو در مفصلهای لگن

harness
Spreizhose
قنداق ارتوپدی نوزاد

At the pediatrician
Troubles/development

Beim Kinderarzt
Beschwerden/Entwicklung

پیش پزشک کودکان
ناراحتیها / رشد

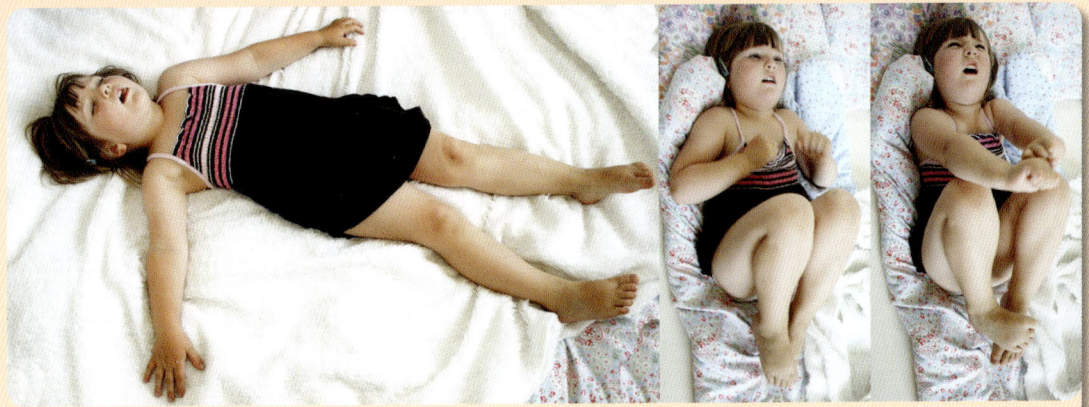

motionless
regungslos
بی تحرک

twitch/spasms
Zuckungen/Krämpfe
تشنج / گرفتگی عضله ها

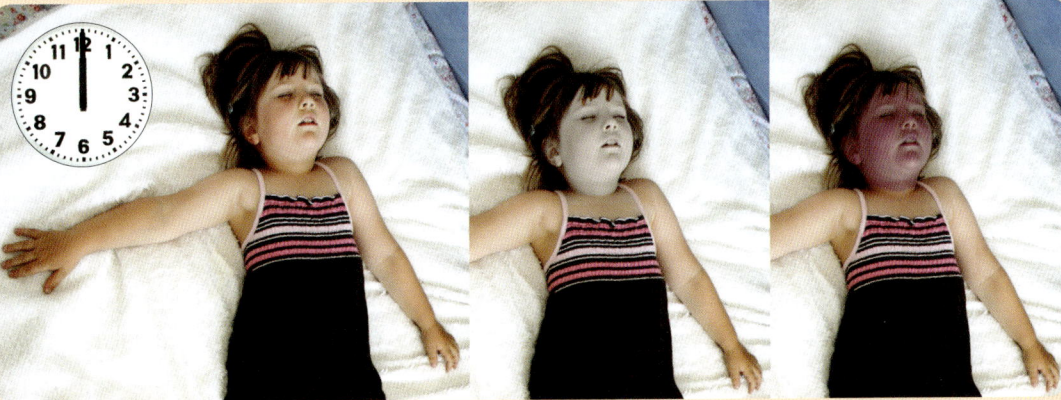

How long?
Wie lange?
چه مدت؟

complexion
Gesichtsfarbe
رنگ صورت

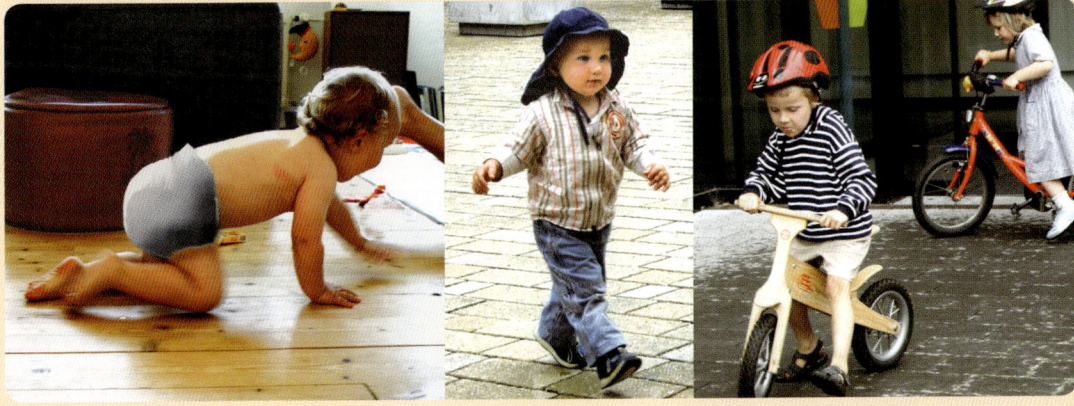

crawling
Krabbeln
چهاردست و پا راه رفتن

walking
Laufen
راه رفتن

agility/exercise
Bewegung
حرکت

At the pediatrician / Beim Kinderarzt
Development/behavior / Entwicklung/Verhalten

پیش پزشک کودکان
رشد / رفتار

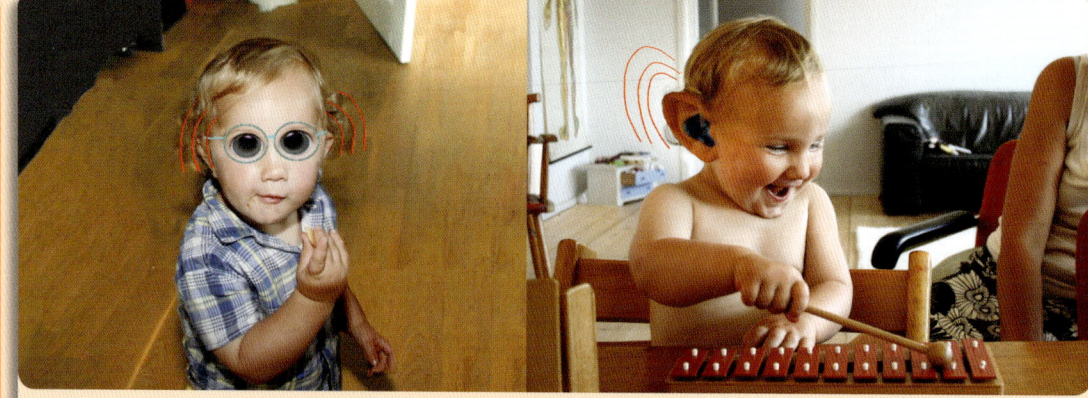

seeing | listening
Sehen | Hören
دیدن | شنیدن

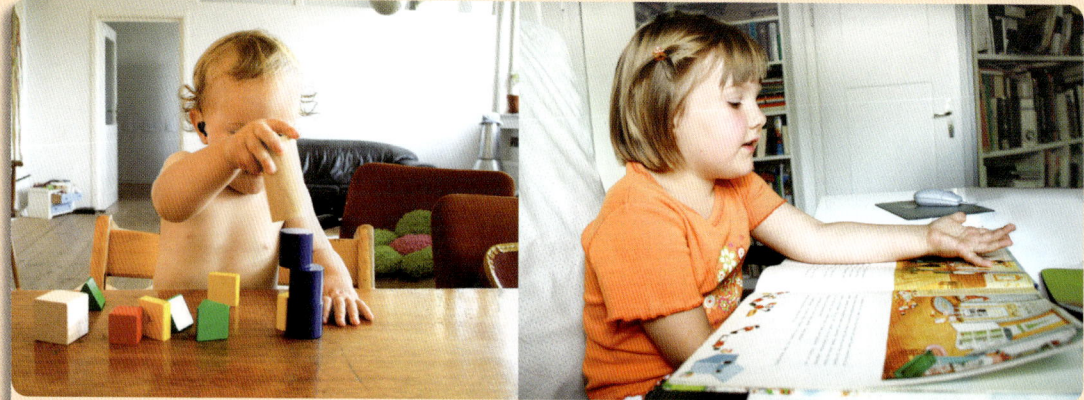

Can the child focus on one issue for a relatively long time?
Kann sich das Kind längere Zeit konzentriert mit einer Sache beschäftigen?
آیا بچه شما میتواند مدت زیادی سرگرم یک چیز باشد؟

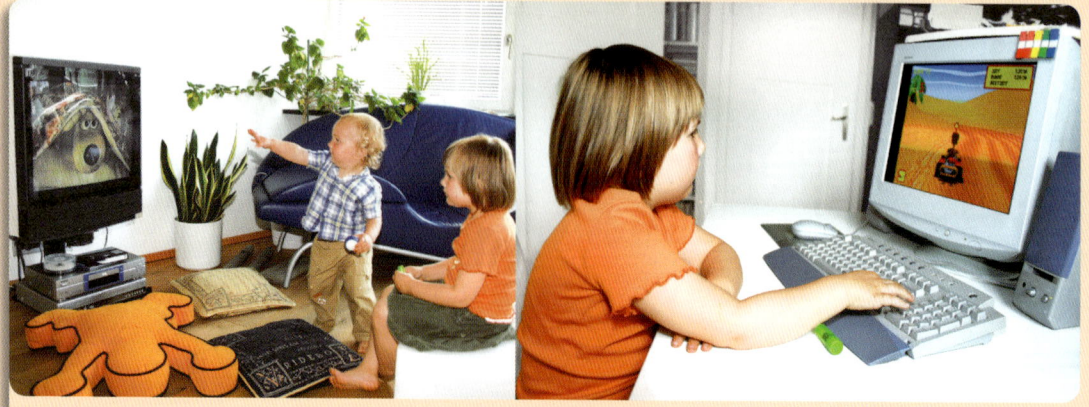

television | computer
Fernseher | Computer
تلویزیون | کامپیوتر

At the pediatrician
Diseases

Beim Kinderarzt
Krankheiten

پیش پزشک کودکان
بیماریها

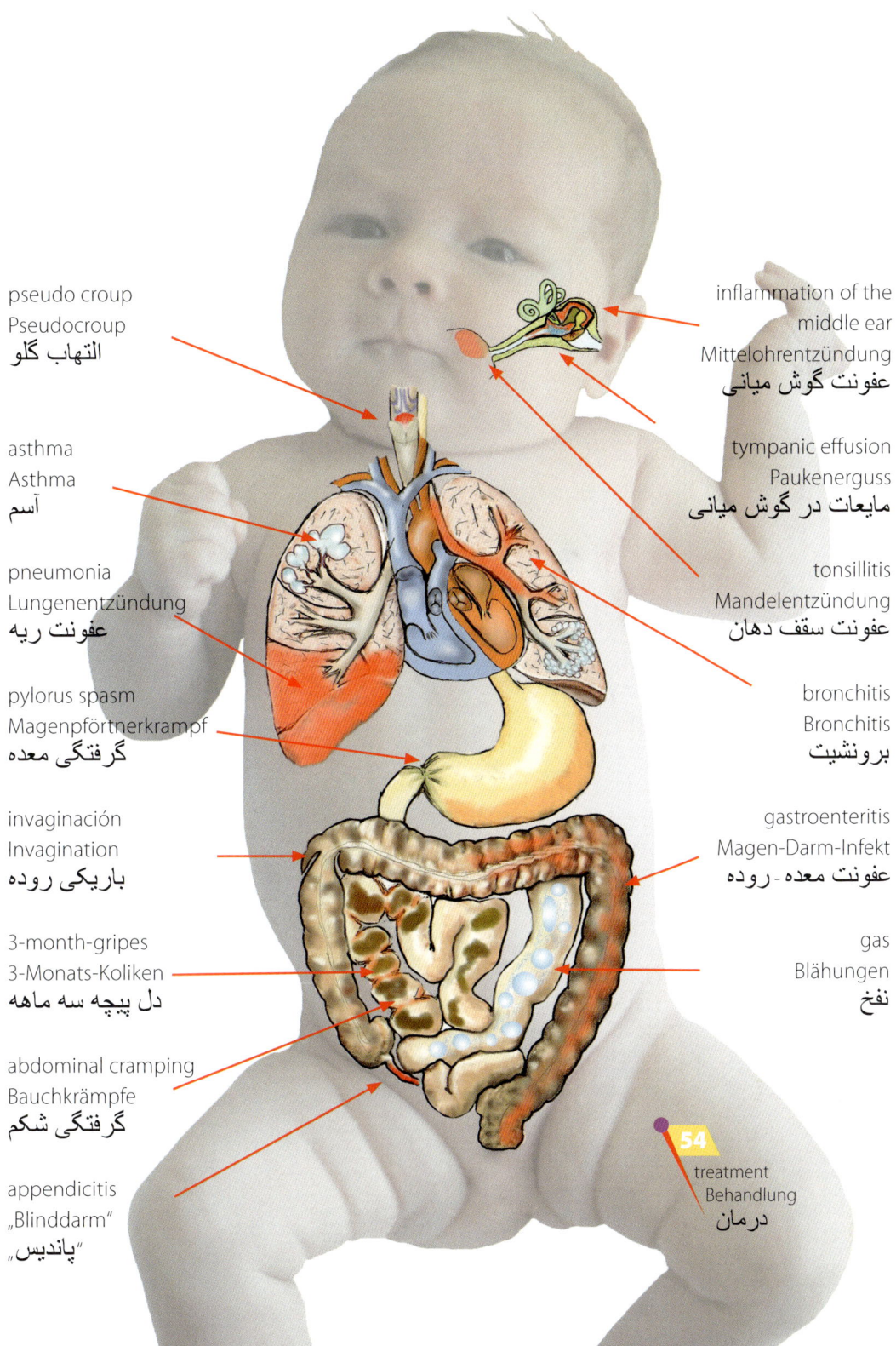

pseudo croup
Pseudocroup
التهاب گلو

asthma
Asthma
آسم

pneumonia
Lungenentzündung
عفونت ریه

pylorus spasm
Magenpförtnerkrampf
گرفتگی معده

invaginación
Invagination
باریکی روده

3-month-gripes
3-Monats-Koliken
دل پیچه سه ماهه

abdominal cramping
Bauchkrämpfe
گرفتگی شکم

appendicitis
„Blinddarm"
„پاندیس"

inflammation of the middle ear
Mittelohrentzündung
عفونت گوش میانی

tympanic effusion
Paukenerguss
مایعات در گوش میانی

tonsillitis
Mandelentzündung
عفونت سقف دهان

bronchitis
Bronchitis
برونشیت

gastroenteritis
Magen-Darm-Infekt
عفونت معده - روده

gas
Blähungen
نفخ

54
treatment
Behandlung
درمان

At the gynecologist
Troubles

Beim Frauenarzt
Beschwerden

پیش پزشک زنان
ناراحتیها

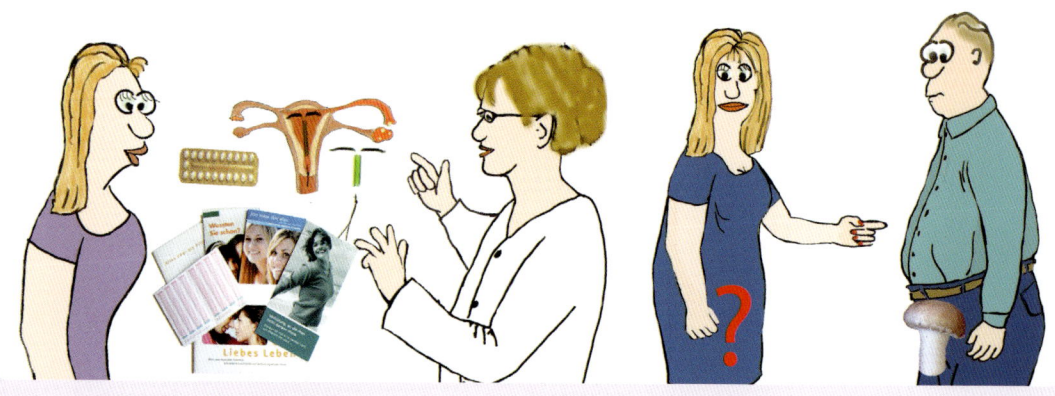

information/birth control: pill, I.U.D
Information/Verhütung: Pille, Spirale
اطلاعات/پیشگیری حاملگی: قرص ضد حاملگی آی - یو دی

partner examination/sexual transmitted disease?
Partneruntersuchung/Geschlechtskrankheit?
معاینه همسر / بیماری جنسی؟

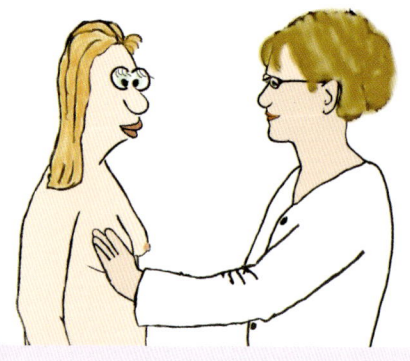
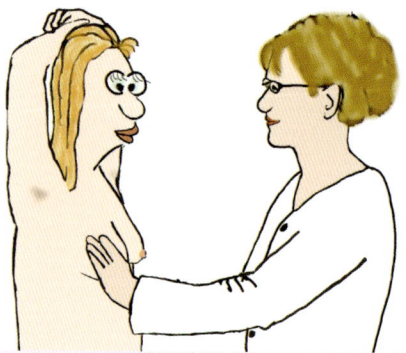

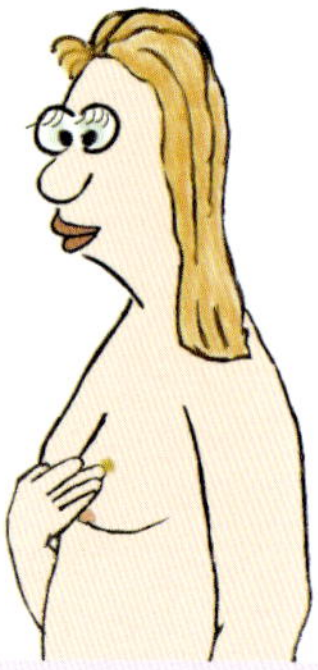

preventive check, digital examination
Brustkrebsvorsorge, Tastuntersuchung
پیشگیری بوسیله معاینه لمسی

node
Knoten
گره ها

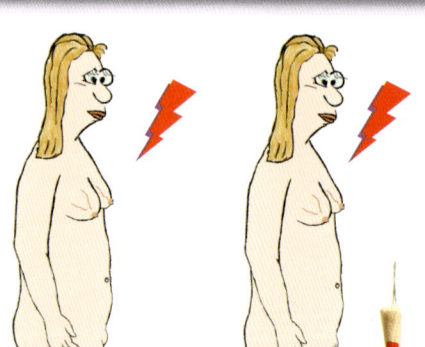
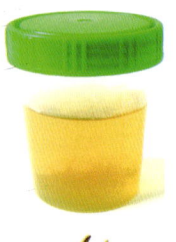
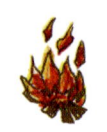
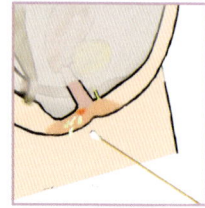

urologist
Urologe
پزشک ارولوژ

tearing pain of the breast
before   during the period
Ziehen der Brust
vor der Periode   während der Periode
سینه درد قبل از پریود / موقع پریود

burning while micturation
Brennen beim Wasserlassen
سوزش هنگام ادرار

discharge/itching
Ausfluss/Juckreiz
ترشح / خارش

At the gynecologist
Troubles/examination

Beim Frauenarzt
Beschwerden/Untersuchung

پیش پزشک زنان
ناراحتیها / معاینه

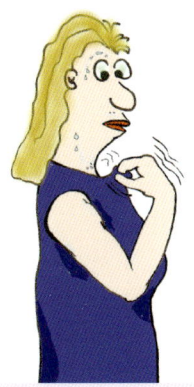
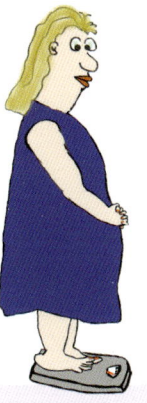
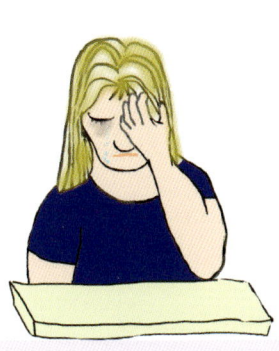

„menopause":　　hot flushes　　　　hair loss　　　increase in weight　　depressions
„Wechseljahre":　Hitzewallungen　　Haarausfall　　Gewichtszunahme　　Depressionen
"دوران یائسگی"　احساس گرمای ناگهانی　ریزش مو　افزایش وزن　افسردگی

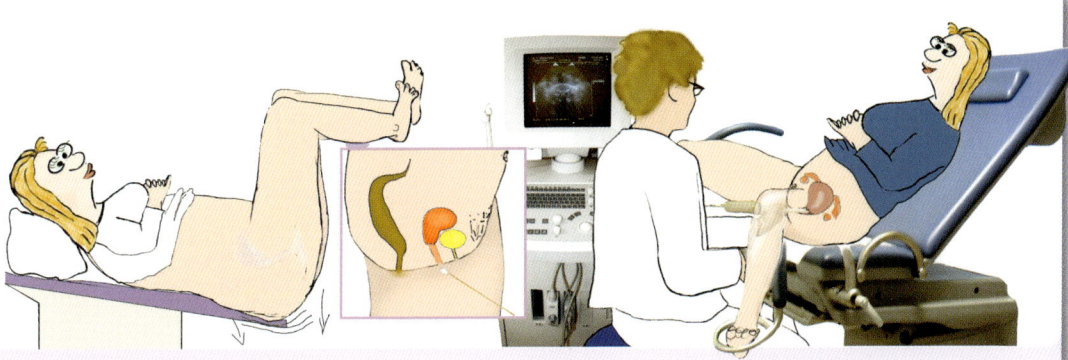

relax your bottom　smear test –　　　　　　　　　ultrasound of the lower body
　　　　　　　　　from the mouth of the uterus
Po locker lassen　Abstrich – Muttermund　　　　Ultraschall Unterleib
باسن را شل کنید　آزمایش ترشحات دهانه رحم　　سونوگرافی زیر شکم

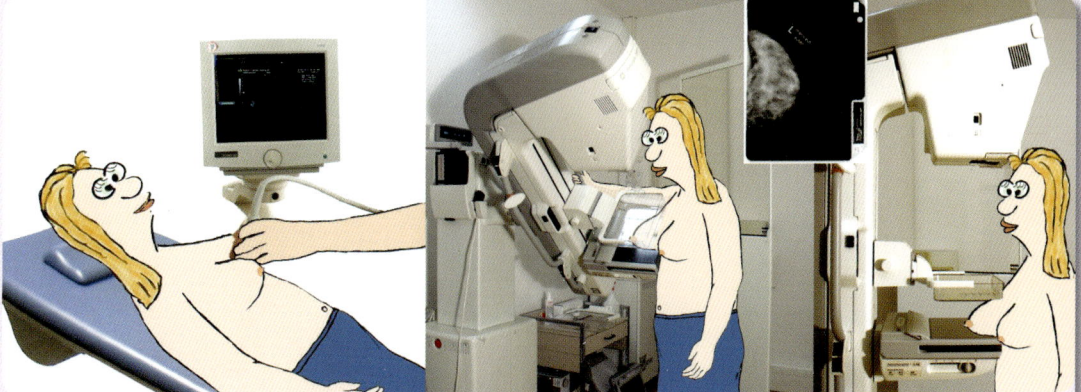

ultrasound breast　　　　　　　mammography
Ultraschall Brust　　　　　　　Mammographie
سونوگرافی سینه　　　　　　　رادیولوژی سینه

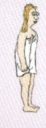

At the gynecologist
Questions

Beim Frauenarzt
Fragen

پیش پزشک زنان
سوال‌ها

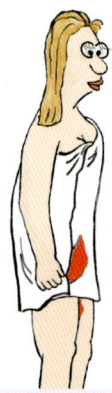
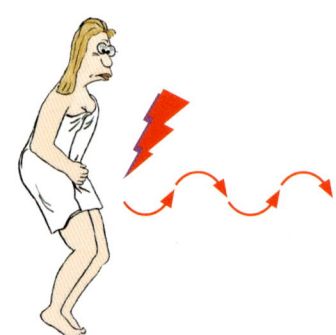
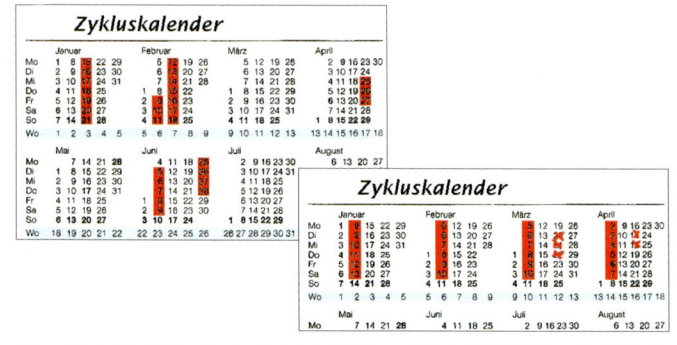

date • Datum: _ _ . _ _ . _ _ _ _   : تاریخ

last period	duration	menstruation cycle	amenorrhoea
letzte Periode	Dauer	Zykluskalender	keine Periode
آخرین پریود	مدت زمان	دوره گردش	بدون پریود

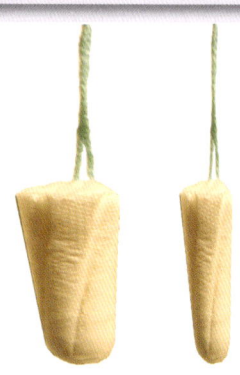
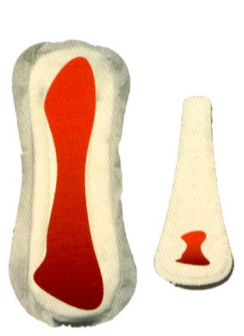

cramps/pain	irregular bleeding	spotting
Krämpfe/Schmerz	Blutungen unregelmäßig	Zwischenblutungen
گرفتگی عضلات / درد	خونریزی نامرتب	خونریزی میان دوره ای

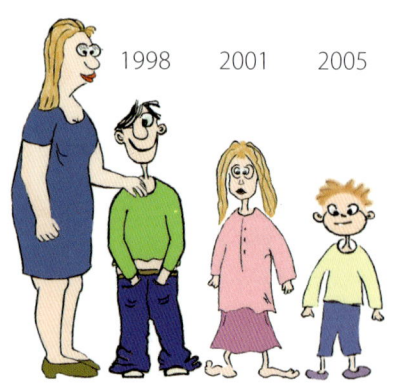

1998 2001 2005

bleeding weak/heavy		children
Blutung schwach/stark		Kinder
خونریزی کم / زیاد		بچه ها

34

At the gynecologist
Questions/troubles

Beim Frauenarzt
Fragen/Beschwerden

پیش پزشک زنان
سوالها / ناراحتیها

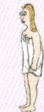

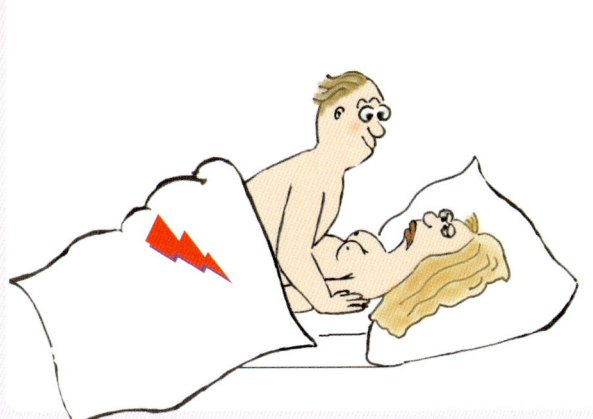

painful sexual intercourse
Schmerzen Geschlechtsverkehr
درد هنگام آمیزش جنسی

dry vagina
trockene Scheide
خشک بودن آلت تناسلی خانمها

interest yes/no
Lust ja/nein
هوس بله / نه

35

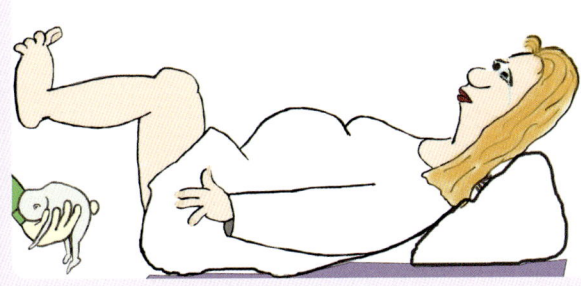

miscarriage – what month?
Fehlgeburt – welcher Monat?
سقط جنین – چند ماهگی؟

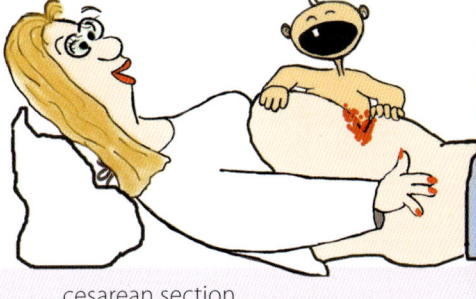

cesarean section
Kaiserschnitt
سزارین

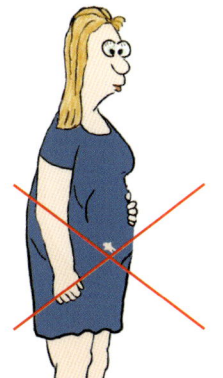

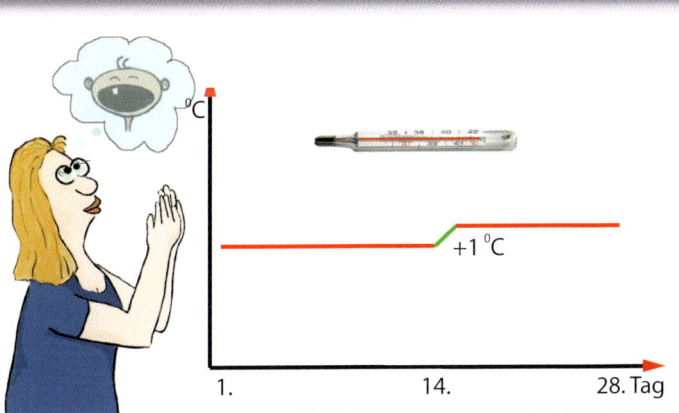

abortion?
Abtreibung?
کورتاژ؟

desire of children
Kinderwunsch
آرزوی بچه

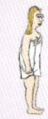

At the gynecologist
Troubles

Beim Frauenarzt
Beschwerden

پیش پزشک زنان
ناراحتیها

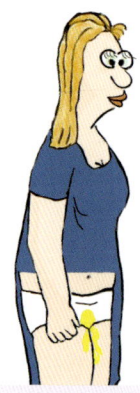 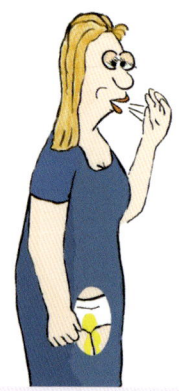 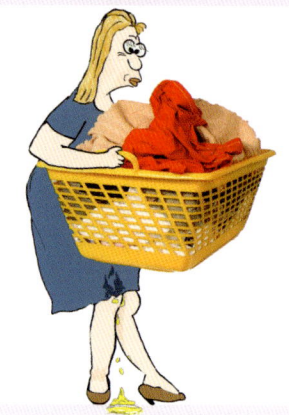

incontinence
Blasenschwäche
عدم کنترل ادرار

when coughing
beim Husten
عدم کنترل ادرار هنگام سرفه کردن

when lifting
beim Heben
عدم کنترل ادرار هنگام بلند کردن

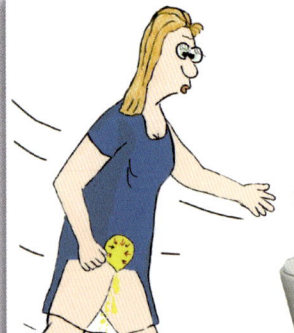 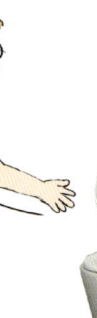

with urge
mit Harndrang
با فشار ادرار

loss of water while lying
Urinverlust im Liegen
عدم کنترل ادرار هنگام خواب

when getting up
beim Aufstehen
هنگام برخاستن

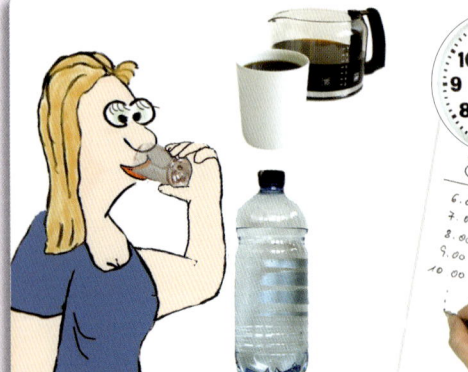 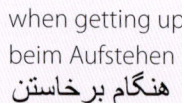 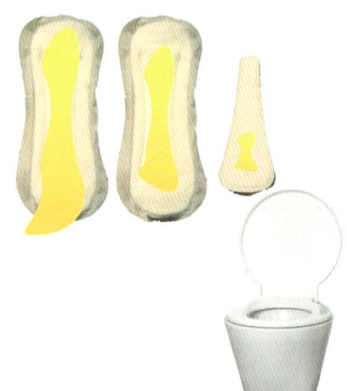

write down: volumen and time of drinking, voiding, pads
Protokoll führen: Trinken, Wasser lassen, Vorlagen
یادداشت کنید: نوشیدن، ادرار کردن، نمونه ها

How many pads?
Wie viel Vorlagen?
چند نمونه؟

At the gynecologist
Examination/treatment

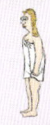

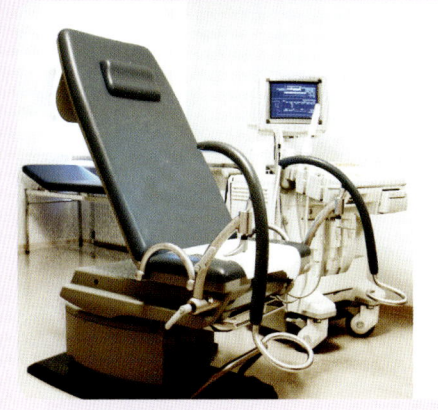

Beim Frauenarzt
Untersuchung/Therapie

پیش پزشک زنان
معاینه / درمان

examination chair
Untersuchungsstuhl
صندلی معاینه

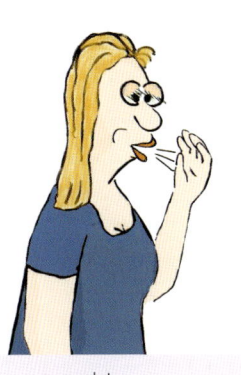

cough!
husten!
سرفه کنید!

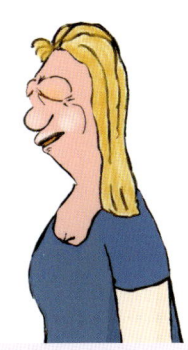

press!
pressen!
فشار دهید!

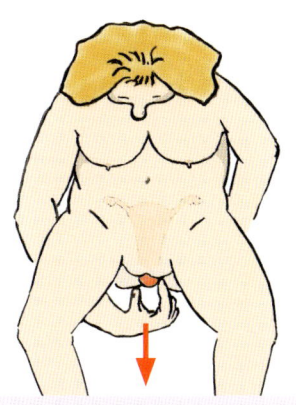

uterine descent
Gebärmuttersenkung
پائین آوردن رحم

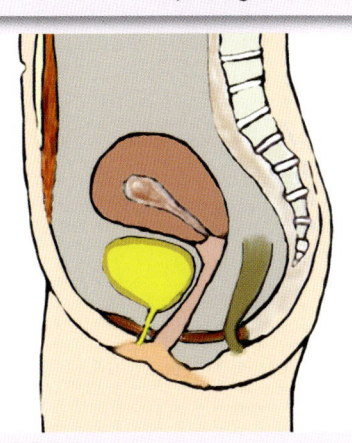

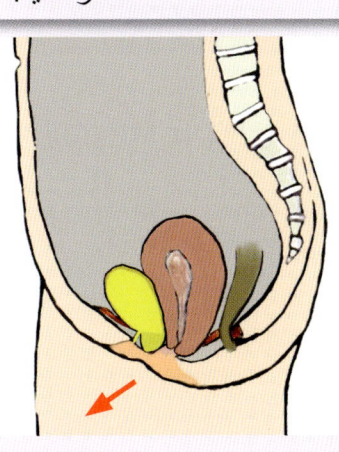

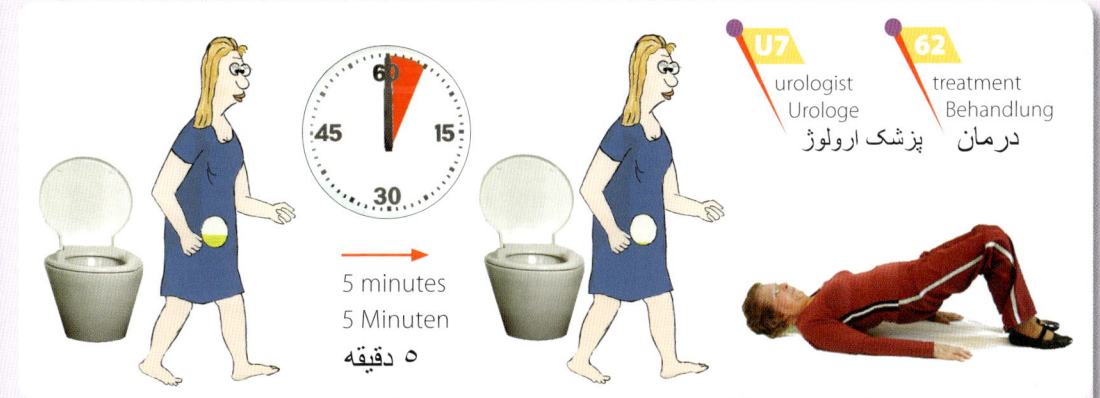

U7 urologist
Urologe
پزشک ارولوژ

62 treatment
Behandlung
درمان

5 minutes
5 Minuten
۵ دقیقه

passing water 2 times in a row
2 x hintereinander Wasserlassen
۲ بار پشت سر هم ادرار کنید

pelvic floor gymnastic
Beckenbodengymnastik
ژیمناستیک درازکش

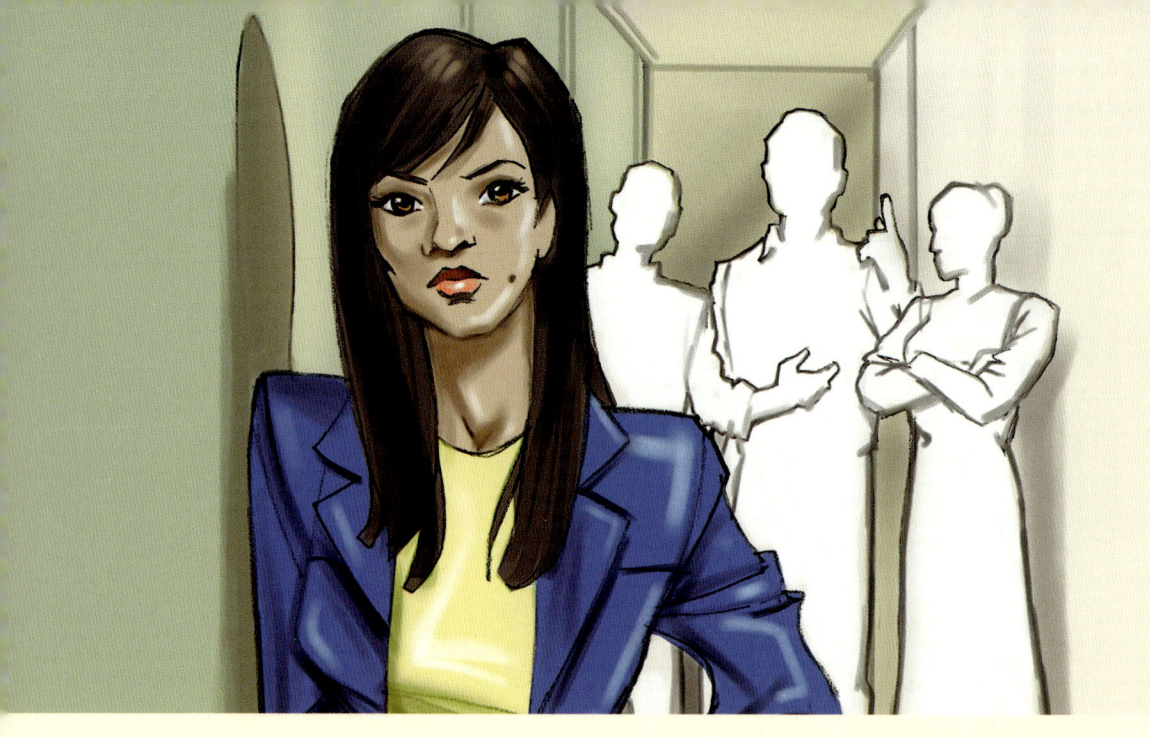

Illustration: © Michael Meier

Du entscheidest, wen und wann Du heiratest!

Informationen finden Sie unter: www.zwangsheirat.de und www.integrationsbeauftragter.de

TERRE DES FEMMES -
Menschenrechte für die
Frau e.V.

Baden-Württemberg
DER INTEGRATIONSBEAUFTRAGTE DER LANDESREGIERUNG

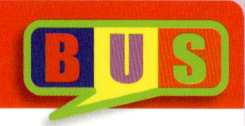

BUS
Bild und Sprache e.V.

Eine Sprache zu lernen ist viel einfacher in der Wort-Bild-Kombination. Wir unterstützen die Entwicklung von Materialien, mit denen man sich schnell und unkompliziert einfache medizinische Begriffe aneignen oder sich im Notfall auch sprachunabhängig über Bilder beim Arzt oder mit der Schwester verständigen kann.

www.medi-bild.de

Forum für eine kultursensible Altenhilfe

Die Institutionen der Altenhilfe stehen vor der Herausforderung, das Recht alt gewordener MigrantInnen auf Beratung, Betreuung und Pflege sicherzustellen und ihre Angebote kultursensibel auszurichten. Das bedeutet, sich mit den Bedürfnissen Zugewanderter, deren Sprache und Kultur, ihren Ess- und Lebensgewohnheiten und religiösen Bräuchen auseinander zu setzen. Interkulturelle Kompetenzen sind dabei unabdingbar, fachliche Unterstützung ist hierbei hilfreich. Die vielfältigen Angebote des Forums sind eine Bereicherung sowohl für die beteiligten Einrichtungen und Dienste als auch für die zugewanderten SeniorInnen!

Sind Sie interessiert?
Dann machen Sie mit! Oder nehmen Sie Kontakt zu uns auf.

Weitere Informationen unter **www.kultursensible-altenhilfe.de**

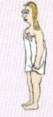

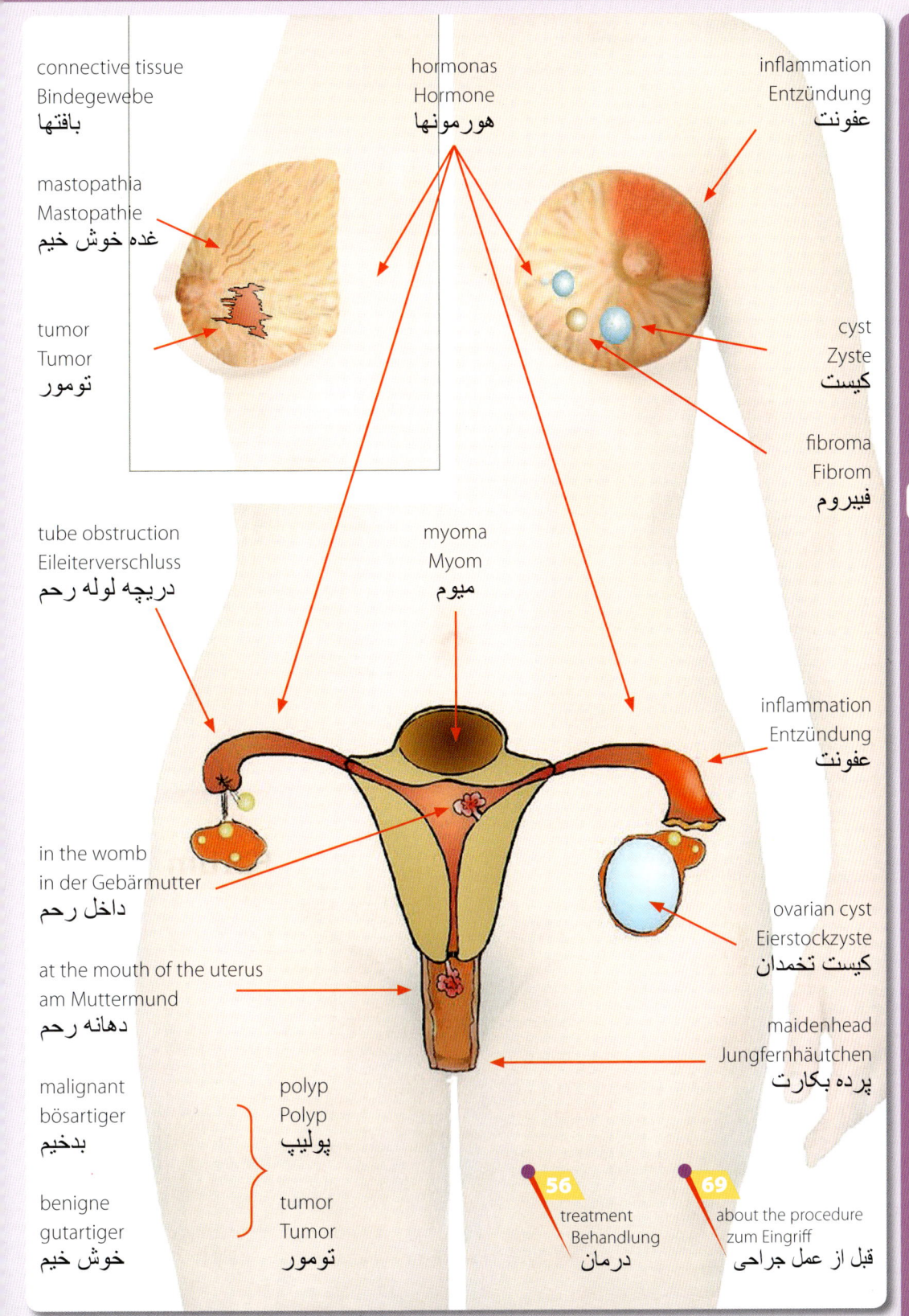

At the gynecologist
Diseases

Beim Frauenarzt
Krankheiten

پیش پزشک زنان
بیماریها

connective tissue Bindegewebe بافتها	hormonas Hormone هورمونها	inflammation Entzündung عفونت
mastopathia Mastopathie غده خوش خیم		cyst Zyste کیست
tumor Tumor تومور		fibroma Fibrom فیبروم
tube obstruction Eileiterverschluss دریچه لوله رحم	myoma Myom میوم	
in the womb in der Gebärmutter داخل رحم		inflammation Entzündung عفونت
at the mouth of the uterus am Muttermund دهانه رحم		ovarian cyst Eierstockzyste کیست تخمدان
malignant bösartiger بدخیم	polyp Polyp پولیپ	maidenhead Jungfernhäutchen پرده بکارت
benigne gutartiger خوش خیم	tumor Tumor تومور	

56 treatment / Behandlung / درمان

69 about the procedure / zum Eingriff / قبل از عمل جراحی

39

At the gynecologist
Pregnancy

Beim Frauenarzt
Schwangerschaft

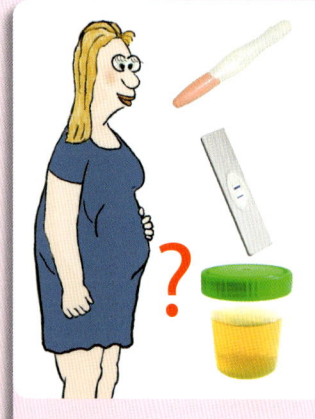

پیش پزشک زنان
حاملگی

pregnancy test	due date	nausea	vomiting
Schwangerschaftstest	Geburtstermin	Übelkeit	Erbrechen
تست حاملگی	وقت زایمان	حالت تهوع	استفراغ

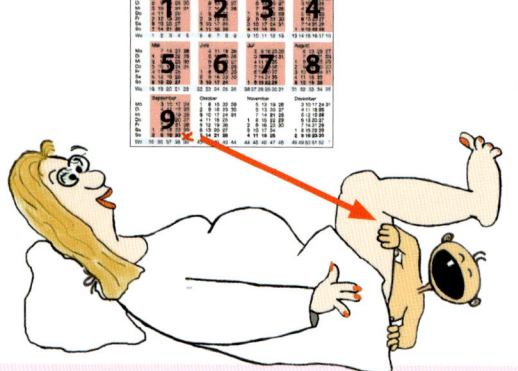

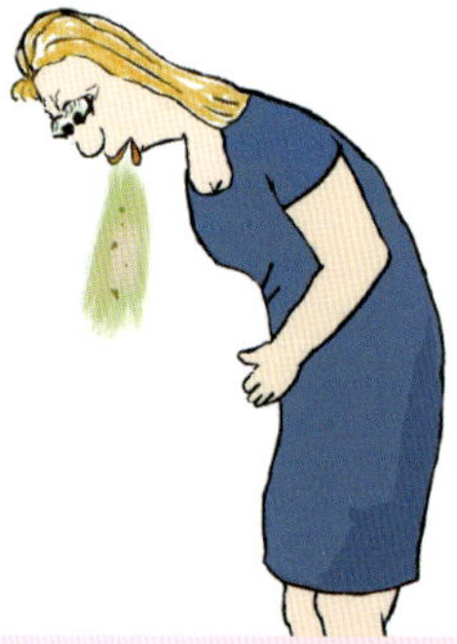

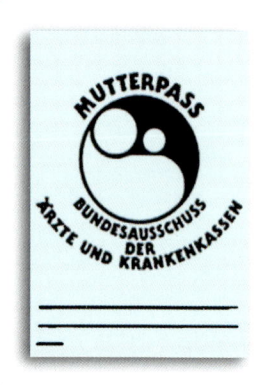

Maternity Card	spotting	secretion/losing liquid
Mutterpass	Blutabgang	Sekret-/Flüssigkeitsabgang
دفترچه مادر	خونریزی	ترشحات / خروج مایعات

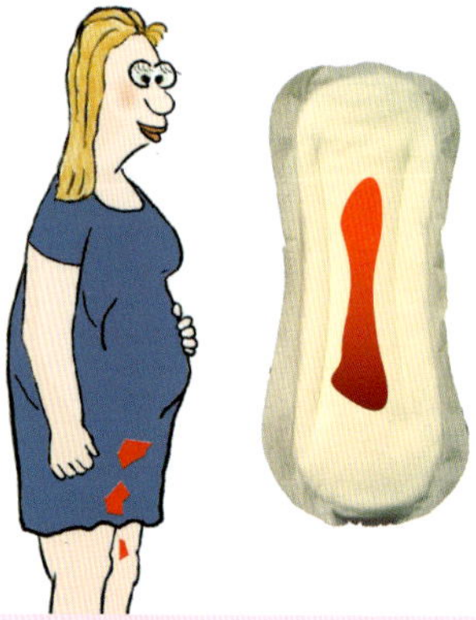

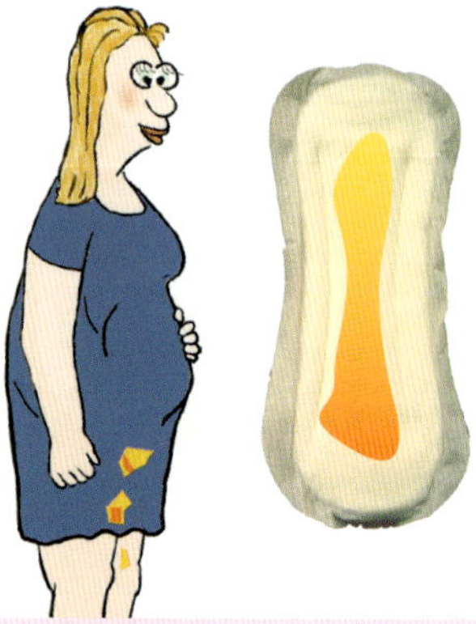

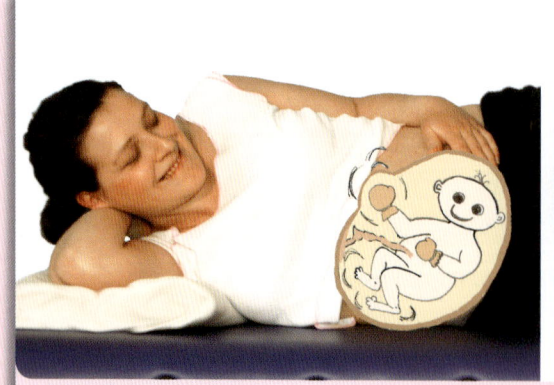

child movement	contraction of the womb/labor pains
Kindsbewegungen	Zusammenziehen der Gebärmutter/Wehen
حرکت جنین	رحم / درد زایمان

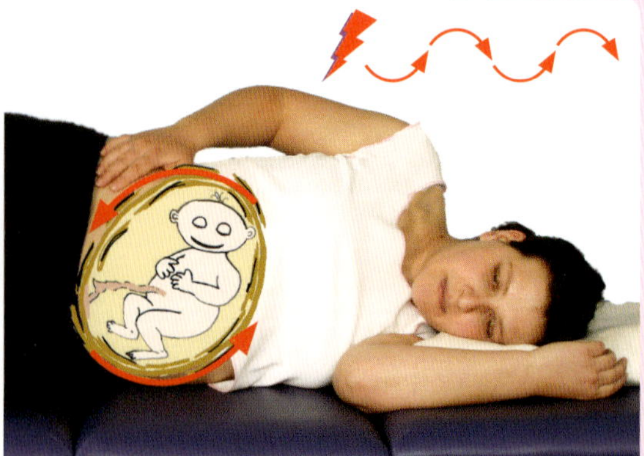

At the gynecologist
Pregnancy

Beim Frauenarzt
Schwangerschaft

پیش پزشک زنان
حاملگی

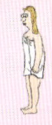

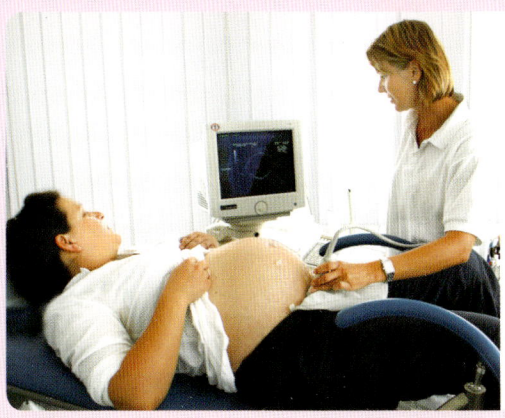

ultrasound
Ultraschall
سونوگرافی

checking growth
Kontrolle Wachstum
کنترل رشد

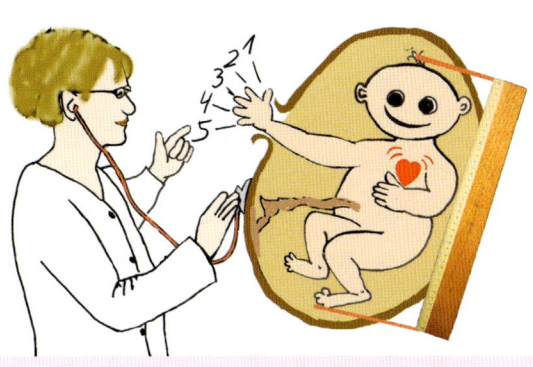

exclusion of abnormality
Ausschluss von Missbildungen
اطمینان از سلامت جنین

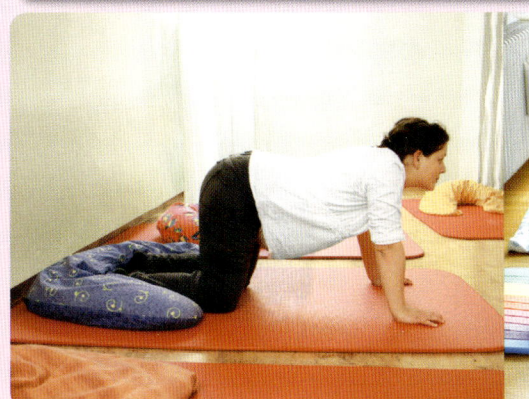

pregnancy exercises
Schwangerschaftsgymnastik
ژیمناستیک دوران حاملگی

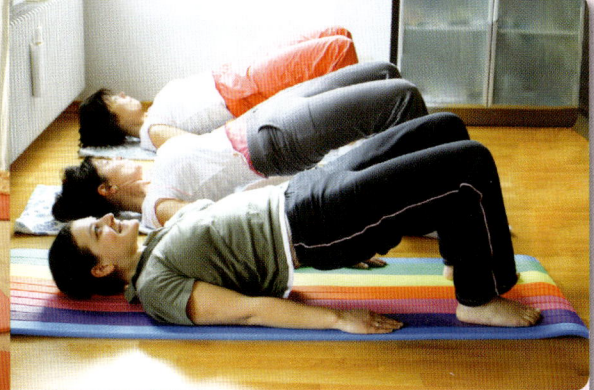

post natal exercises
Rückbildungsgymnastik
ژیمناستیک عضلات پشت

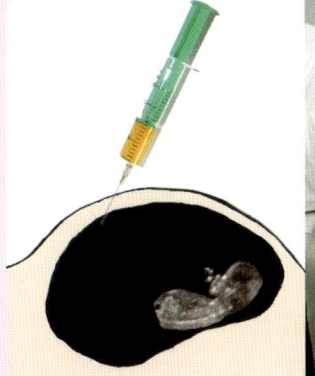

amniocentesis
Fruchtwasseruntersuchung
آزمایش مایع رحم

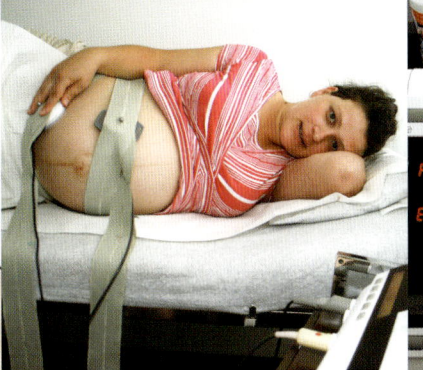

CTG check
CTG Kontrolle
آزمایش سی - تی - جی

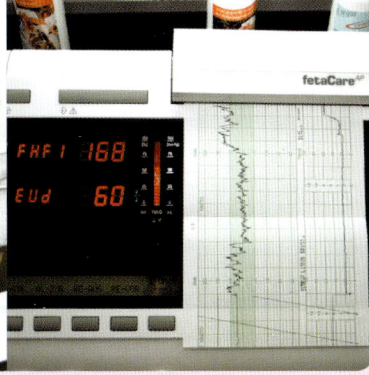

heart sounds/labor
Herztöne/Wehen
ضربان قلب / درد زایمان

| At the orthopedist | Beim Orthopäden | پیش متخصص ارتوپدی |
| Troubles/examination | Beschwerden/Untersuchung | ناراحتیها / معاینه |

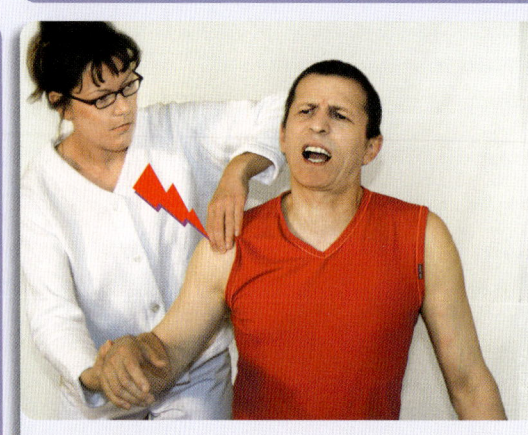

pressure pain
Druckschmerz
درد ناشی از فشار

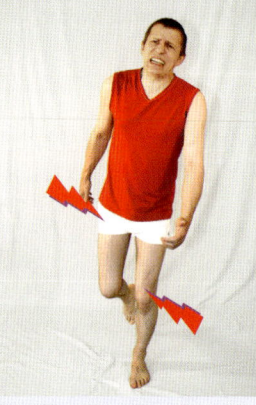

movement pain
Bewegungsschmerz
درد ناشی از حرکت

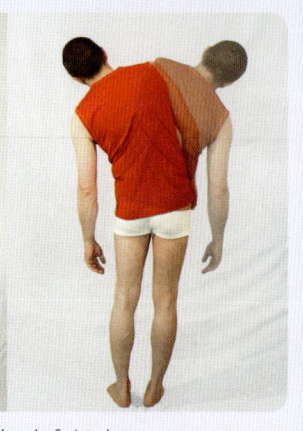

to the left/right
nach links/rechts
به سمت چپ / به سمت راست

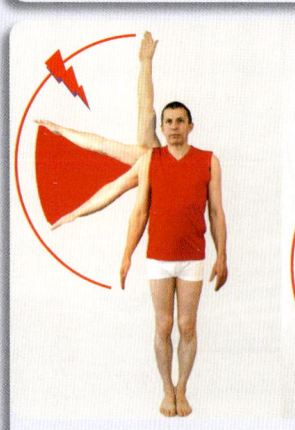

pain from – up to?
Schmerz ab – bis wann?
درد از _ تا کی؟

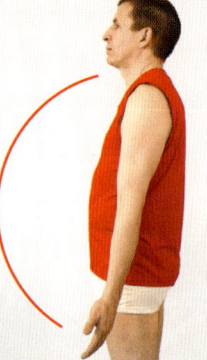

stretch
strecken
کشیدن

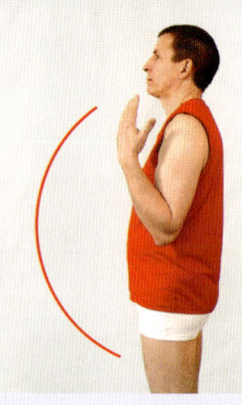

bend
beugen
خم شدن

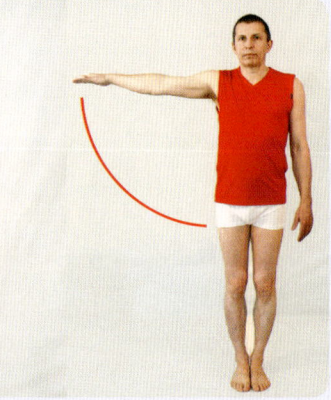

sidewards/to the body
seitwärts/zum Körper
به سمت کنار / به سمت بدن

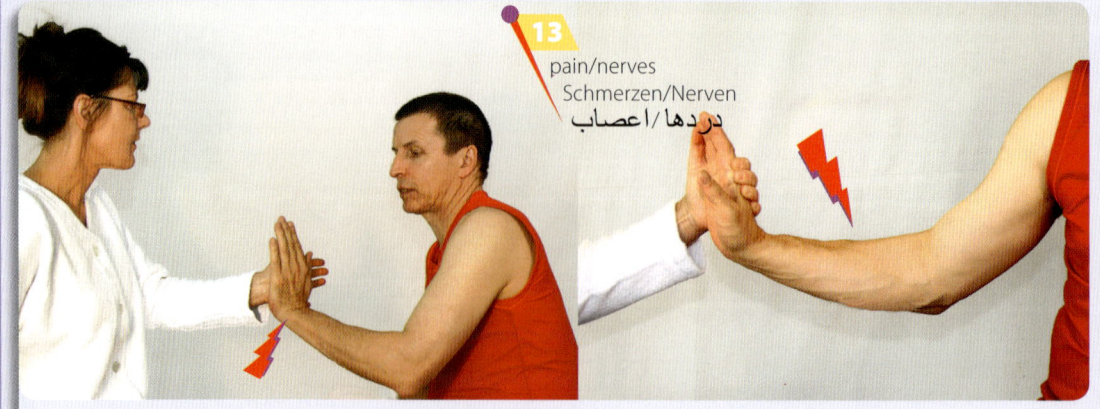

13
pain/nerves
Schmerzen/Nerven
دردها / اعصاب

press hard against it
fest dagegen drücken
محکم فشار دهید

pull back your hand
Hand zurückziehen
دست را بکشید

At the orthopedist
Troubles/examination

Beim Orthopäden
Beschwerden/Untersuchung

پیش متخصص ارتوپدی
ناراحتیها / معاینه

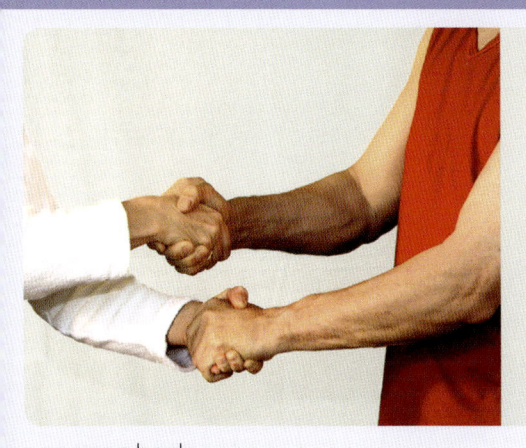

plopp

squeeze hard
fest drücken
کف دست را به سمت بالا / پائین بچرخانید

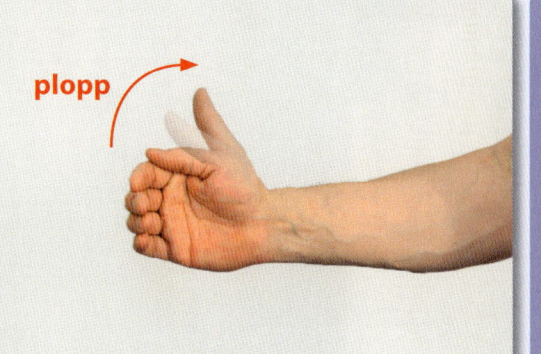

trigger finger
schnellender Finger
حرکت سریع انگشت شصت

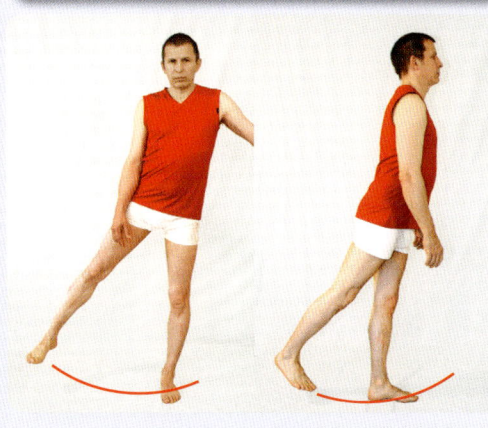

---

sideward – inward – backward – forward
zur Seite – nach innen – hinten – vorne
به سمت کنار ـ داخل ـ پشت ـ جلو

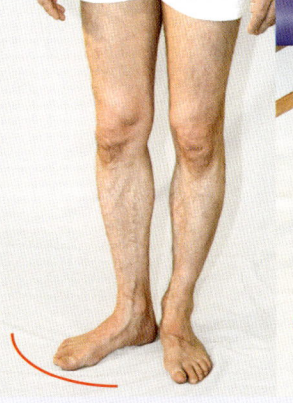

twist the leg
Bein drehen
چرخاندن پا

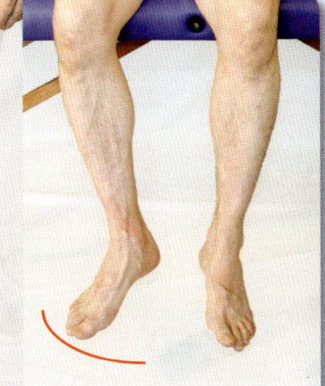

twist the foot
Fuß drehen
چرخاندن کف پا

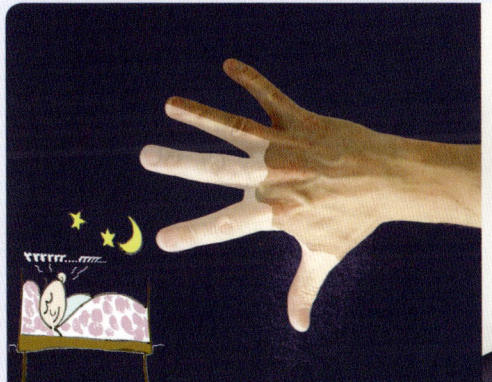

---

numb fingers
Finger schlafen ein
خواب رفتن انگشتها

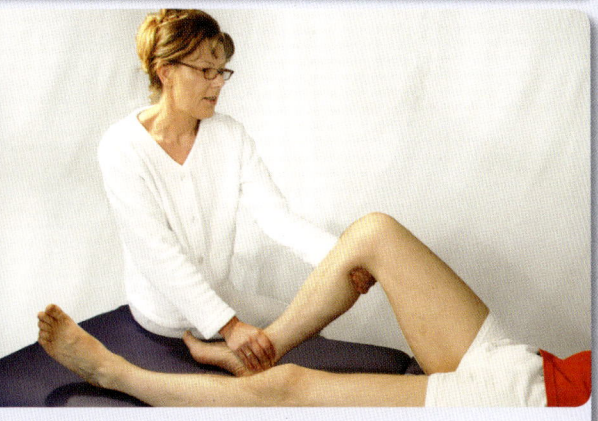

bend – don't do anything else
anwinkeln – sonst nichts machen
خم کردن زانو ـ هیچ کار دیگری نکنید

At the orthopedist
Troubles/examination

Beim Orthopäden
Beschwerden/Untersuchung

پیش متخصص ارتوپدی
ناراحتیها / معاینه

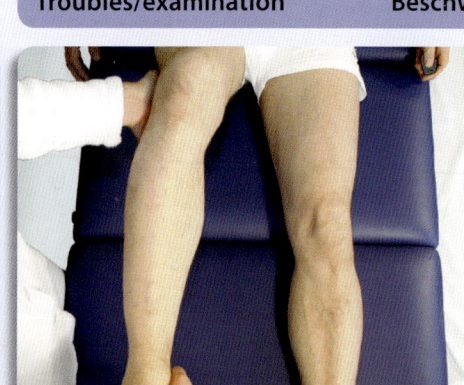

relax
locker lassen
عضلات خود را شل کنید

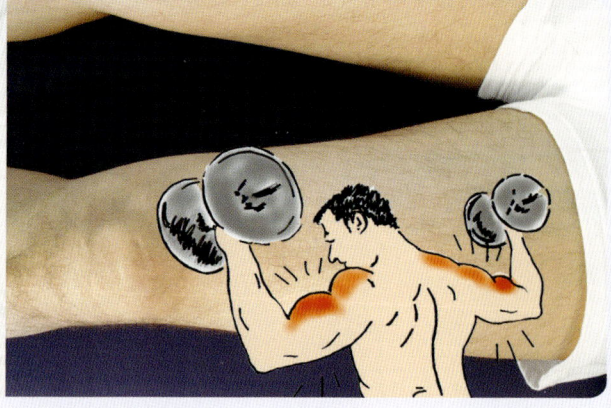

tense the thigh muscles
Oberschenkelmuskulatur anspannen
عضلات ران را سفت کنید.

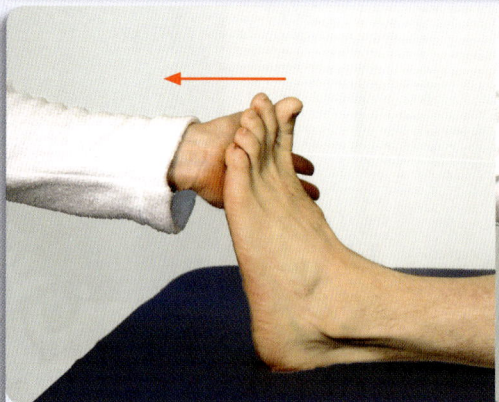

press
drücken
فشار دهید.

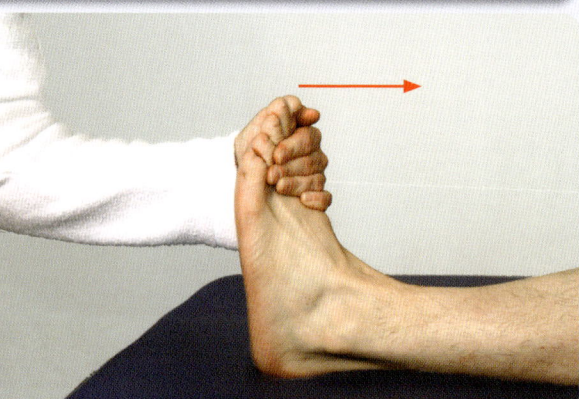

draw the foot
Fuß anziehen
پا را بکشید.

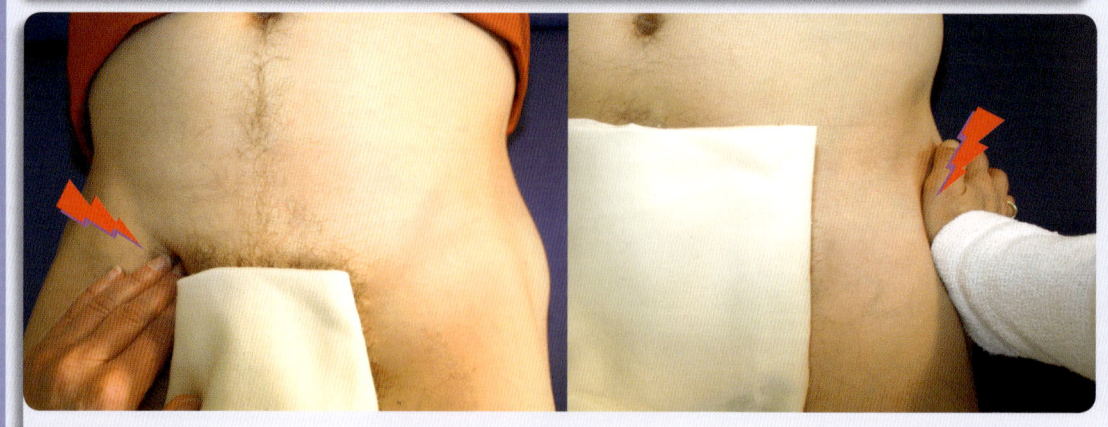

pressure pain of the groin
Leistendruckschmerz
درد روی کشاله ران

knocking pain
Klopfschmerz
درد کوبیدنی

At the orthopedist
Diseases

Beim Orthopäden
Krankheiten

پیش متخصص ارتوپدی
بیماریها

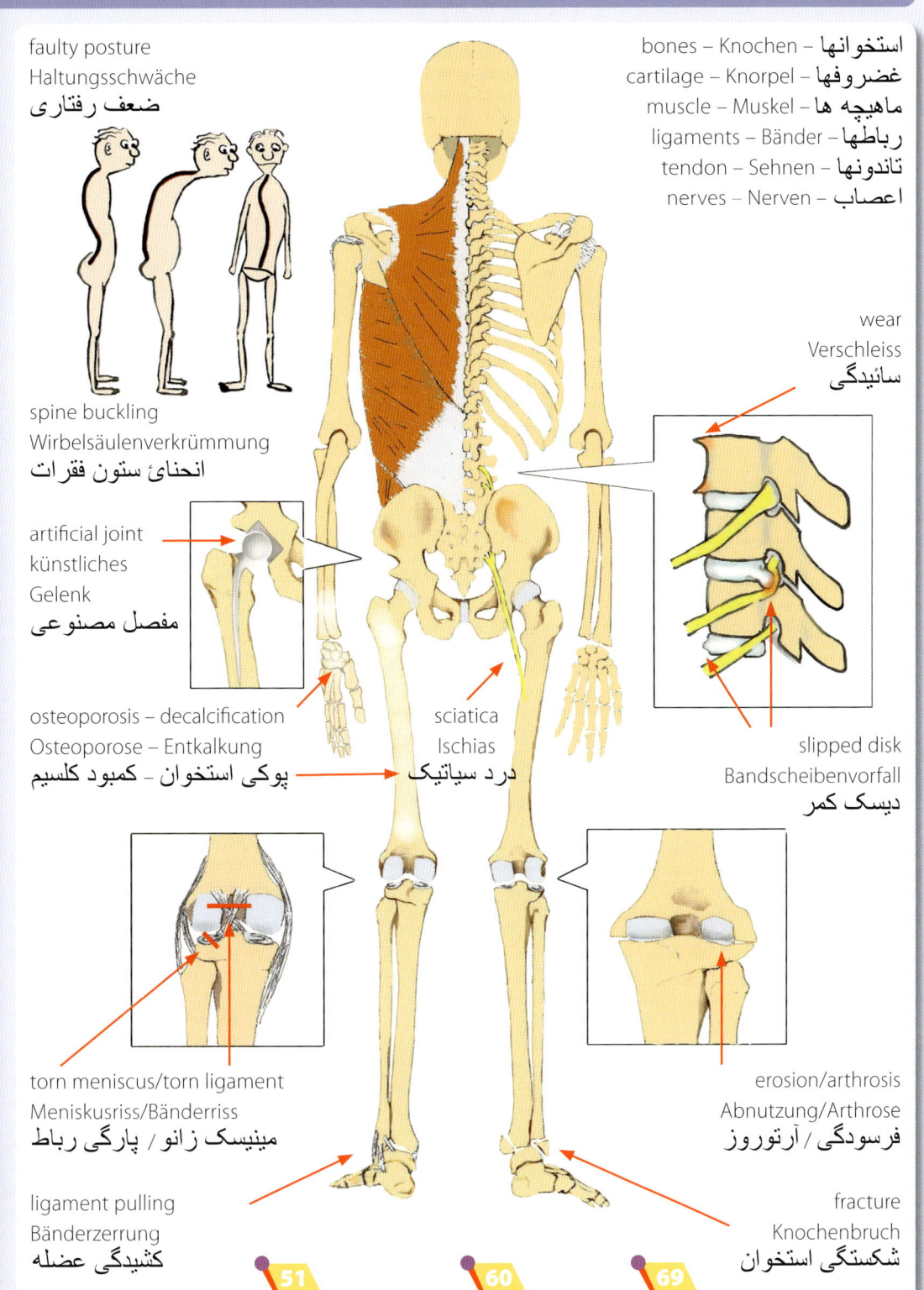

faulty posture
Haltungsschwäche
ضعف رفتاری

bones – Knochen – استخوانها
cartilage – Knorpel – غضروفها
muscle – Muskel – ماهیچه ها
ligaments – Bänder – رباطها
tendon – Sehnen – تاندونها
nerves – Nerven – اعصاب

spine buckling
Wirbelsäulenverkrümmung
انحنائ ستون فقرات

wear
Verschleiss
سائیدگی

artificial joint
künstliches Gelenk
مفصل مصنوعی

osteoporosis – decalcification
Osteoporose – Entkalkung
پوکی استخوان – کمبود کلسیم

sciatica
Ischias
درد سیاتیک

slipped disk
Bandscheibenvorfall
دیسک کمر

torn meniscus/torn ligament
Meniskusriss/Bänderriss
مینیسک زانو / پارگی رباط

erosion/arthrosis
Abnutzung/Arthrose
فرسودگی / آرتروز

ligament pulling
Bänderzerrung
کشیدگی عضله

fracture
Knochenbruch
شکستگی استخوان

51 at the x-raying / beim Röntgen / موقع عکس رادیولوژی

60 treatment / Behandlung / درمان

69 about the procedure / zum Eingriff / قبل از عمل جراحی

45

At the dentist Beim Zahnarzt پیش دندانپزشک

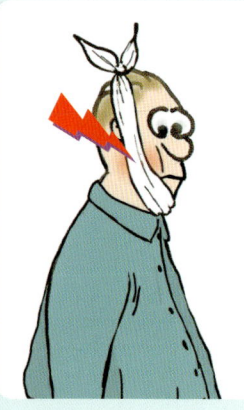

pain	when hot	permanent	when cold	when eating
Zahnschmerzen	bei heiß	dauernd	bei kalt	beim Essen
پیش دندانپزشک	با غذای داغ	همیشه	با غذای سرد	وقت غذا خوردن

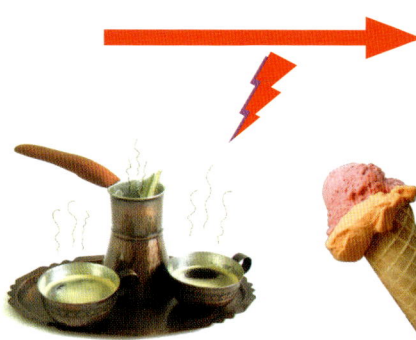

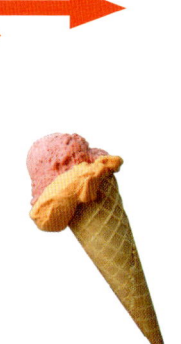

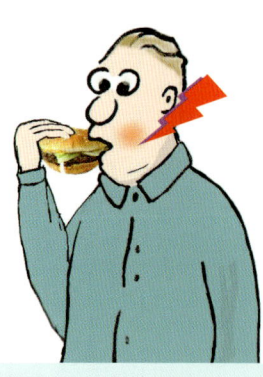

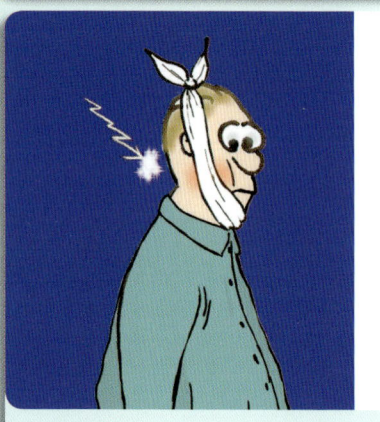

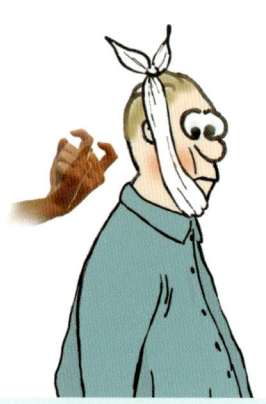

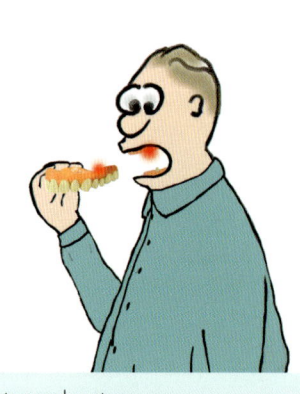

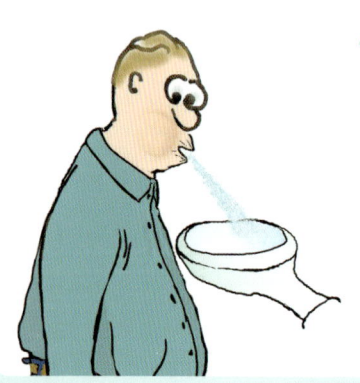

like a flash	throbbing	dentures hurt
blitzartig	pochend	die Prothese drückt
خیلی سریع	ضربه ای	دندان مصنوعی فشار می آورد.

rinse well	injection	pain killers/antibiotic	don´t drink/don´t eat
gut ausspülen	Spritze	Schmerzmittel/Antibiotikum	nichts trinken/~ essen
دهان خود را خوب بشوئید.	آمپول	دارو آنتی بیوتیک	چیزی ننوشید./~نخورید.

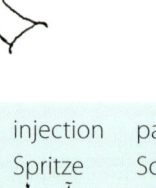

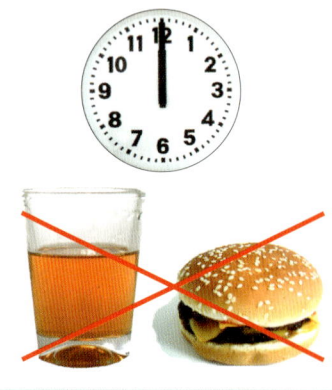

At the dentist / Beim Zahnarzt / پیش دندانپزشک

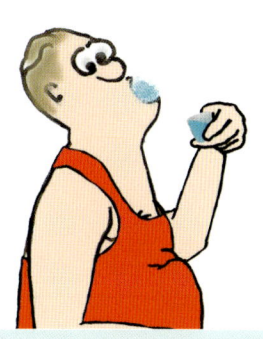

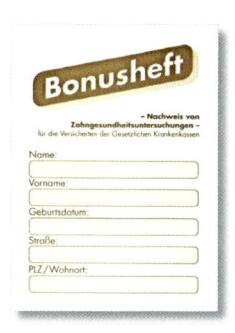

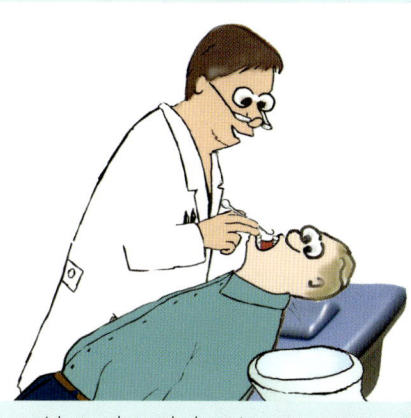

gargle	dental check-up card	control 1-2 times a year/deep dental cleaning
gurgeln	Bonusheft	Kontrolle 1-2 x pro Jahr/professionelle Zahnreinigung
قرقره کردن	پرونده دندانپزشکی	کنترل ۲ بار در سال/ نظافت دندان

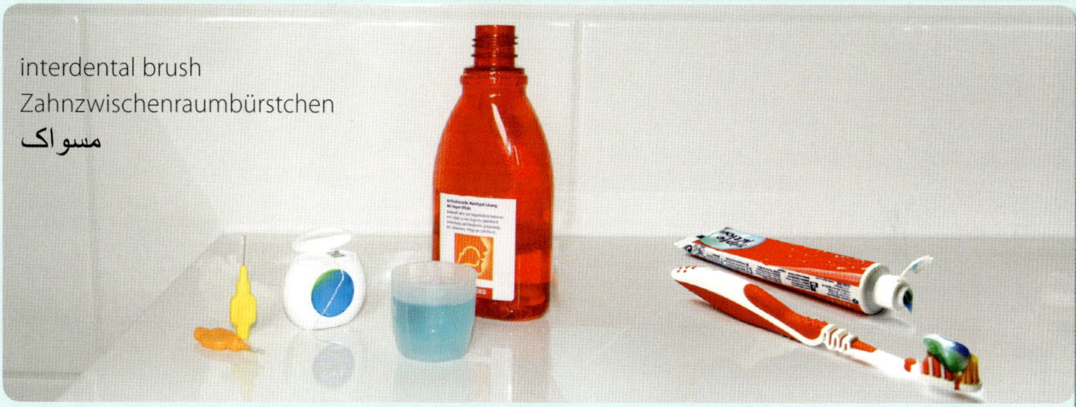

interdental brush
Zahnzwischenraumbürstchen
مسواک

dental care:	floss	mouthwash	toothbrush	toothpaste
Zahnpflege:	Zahnseide	Mundspülung	Zahnbürste	Zahnpasta
نظافت دندان	نخ دندان	شستشوی دهان	مسواک	خمیر دندان

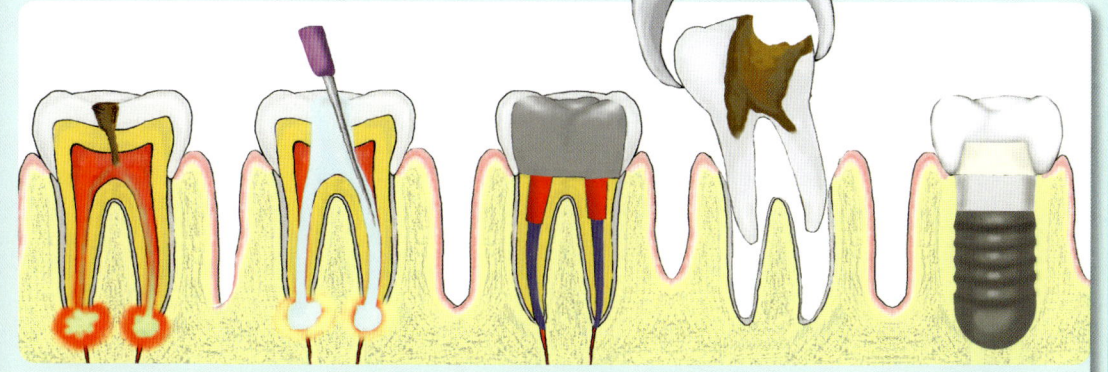

infection	root-canal treatment	with a root pin	extraction	implant
Entzündung	Wurzelbehandlung	mit Wurzelstift	Zahn ziehen	Implantat
عفونت	درمان ریشه دندان	عصب کشی	کشیدن دندان	کاشتن دندان

At the dentist — Beim Zahnarzt — پیش دندانپزشک

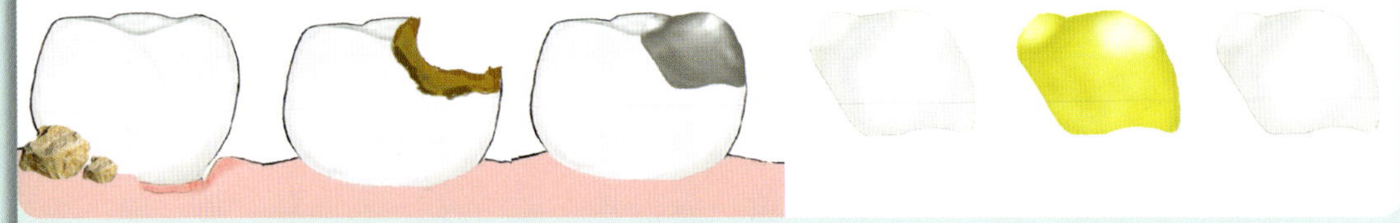

tartar/periodontosis	caries	filling:	amalgam	plastic	inlay gold	porcelain
Zahnstein/Parodontose	Karies	Füllung:	Amalgam	Kunststoff	Inlay Gold	Keramik
جرم دندان/عفونت لثه	پوسیدگی دندان	پر کردن	آمالگام	ماده مصنوعی	طلا	سرامیک

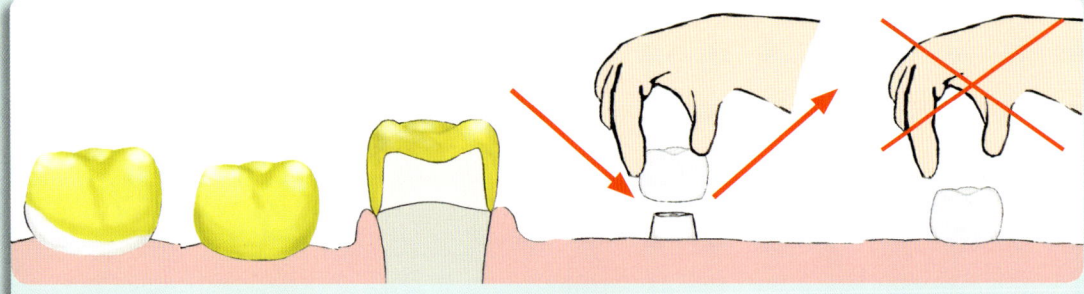

partial crown	crown	temporary	definite crown
Teilkrone	Krone	provisorische	endgültige Krone
نیمه روکش	روکش	موقتی	روکش نهائی

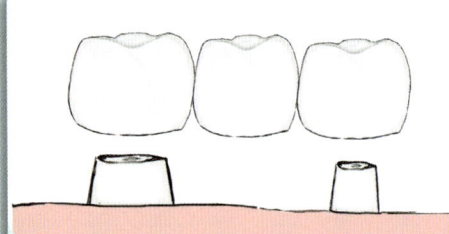

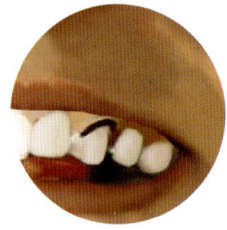

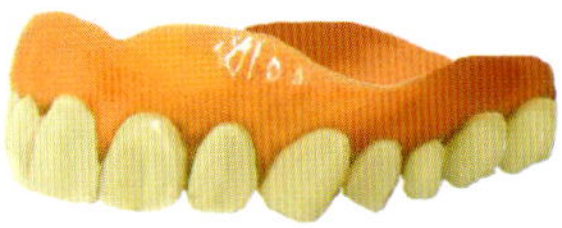

bridge	clasp/partial denture	complete dentures
Brücke	Klammerprothese	Vollprothese
پروتز	پروتز گیره ای	پروتز کامل

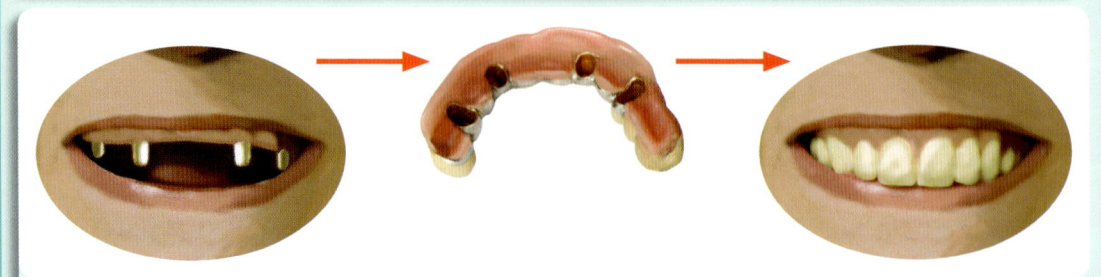

telescope denture
Teleskopprothese
پروتز تلسکوپی

Examination — Untersuchung — معاینه

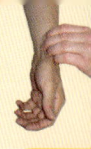

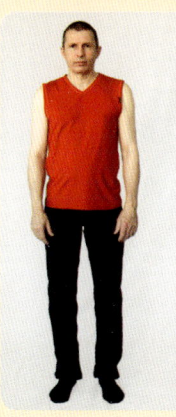

stand up	shirt off/ shirt up	pants down/off	take off all your pants / take everything off
hinstellen	Hemd aus/ Hemd hoch	Hose runter/aus	Unterkörper frei / ganz ausziehen
با یستید.	پیراهن را در بیاورید. / پیراهن را بالا بزنید.	شلوار را پائین بکشید. / شلوار را در بیاورید.	پائین تنه را لخت کنید. / کامل لخت شوید.

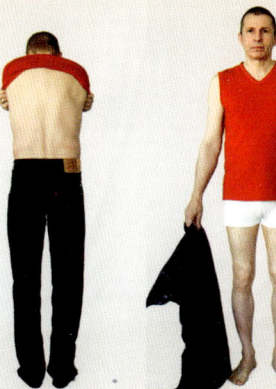

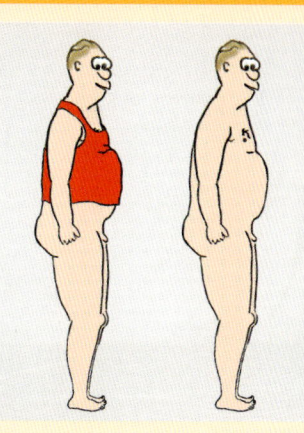

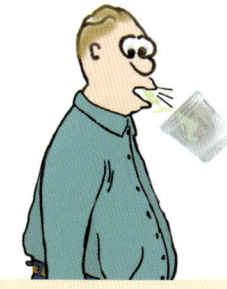

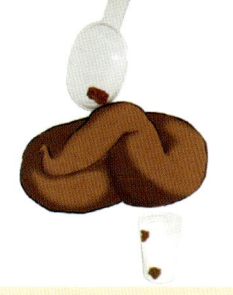

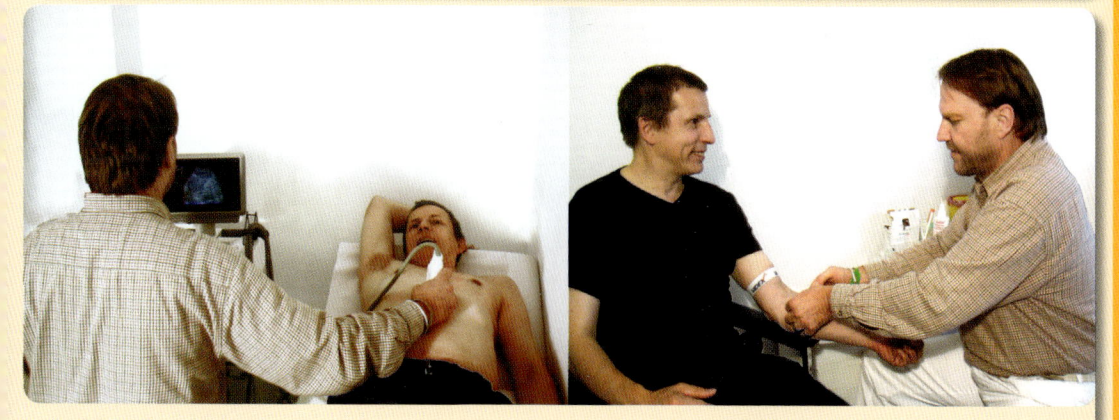

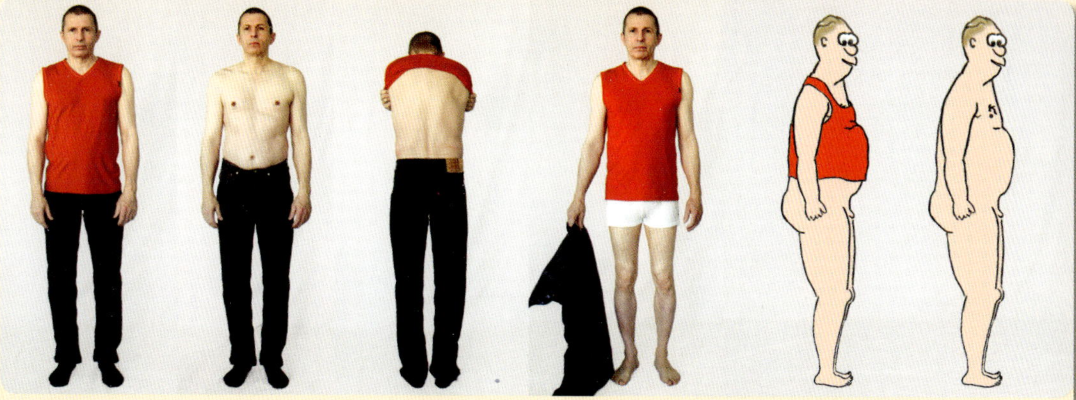

stool sample	urine sample	cough up
Stuhlprobe	Urinprobe	abhusten
آزمایش مدفوع	آزمایش ادرار	سرفه کنید.

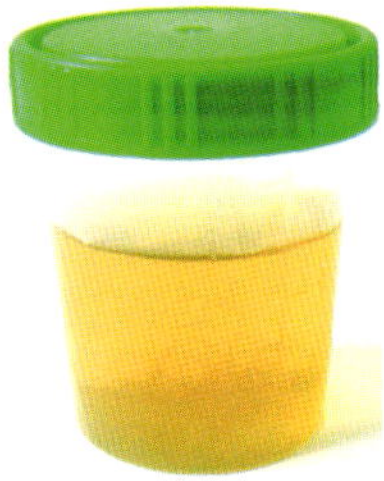

ultrasound	blood sample
Ultraschall	Blutprobe
سونوگرافی	آزمایش خون

49

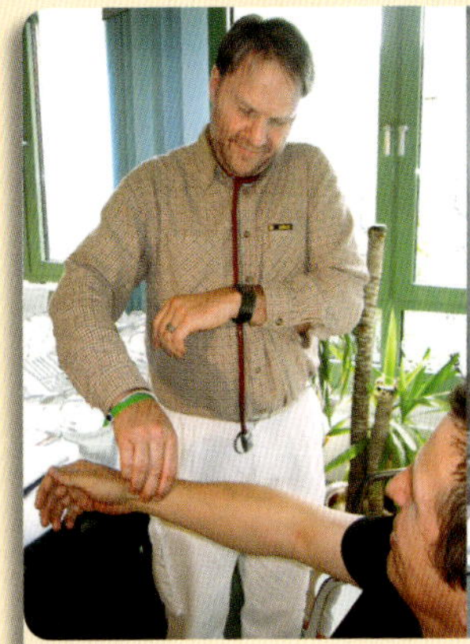

Examination — Untersuchung — معاینه

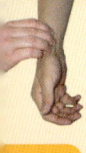

taking the pulse	taking the blood pressure	long-term blood press
Puls messen	Blutdruck messen	Langzeit-Blutdruck
گرفتن نبض	گرفتن فشار خون	فشار خون دائم

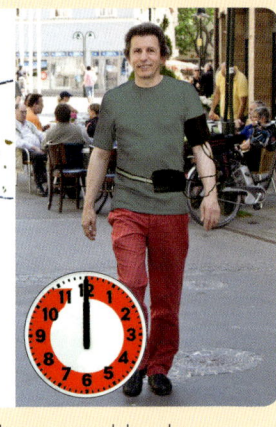

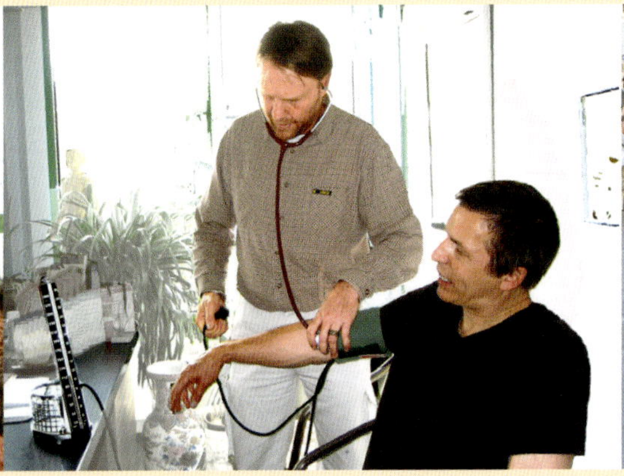

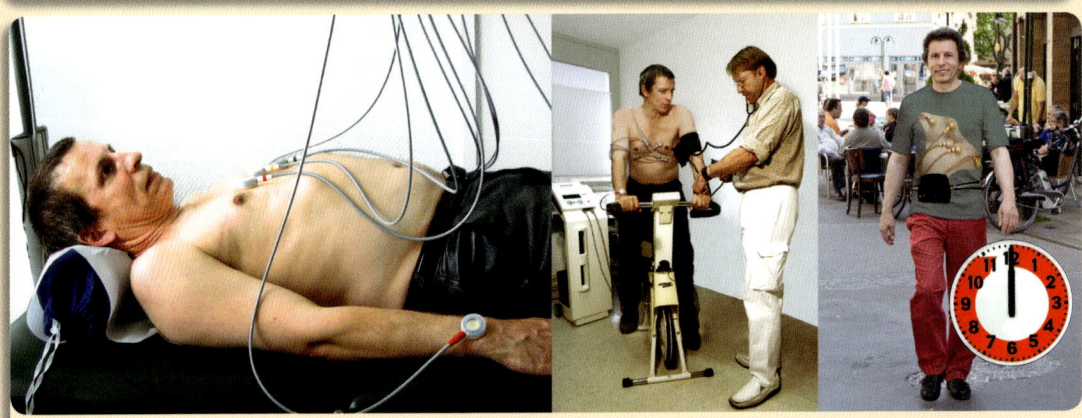

ECG	exercise ECG	long-term ECG
EKG	Belastungs-EKG	Langzeit-EKG
نوار قلب	نوار قلب در حرکت	نوار قلب دائم

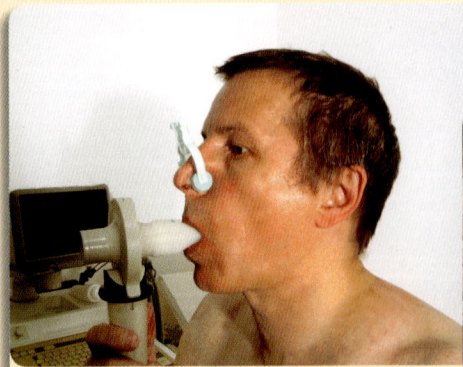

lung function test	breath in	breath out
Lungenfunktionstest	einatmen	ausatmen
آزمایش ریه	نفس بکشید.	نفس را بیرون دهید.

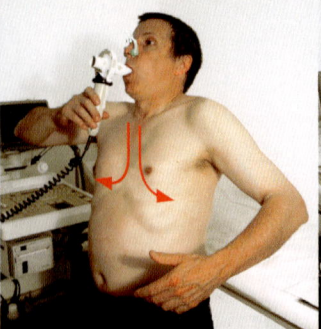

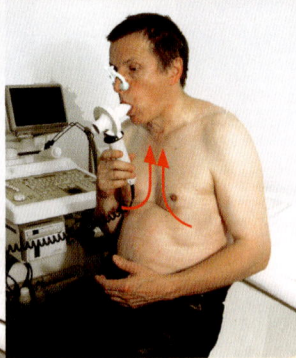

Examination — Untersuchung — معاينه

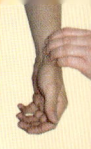

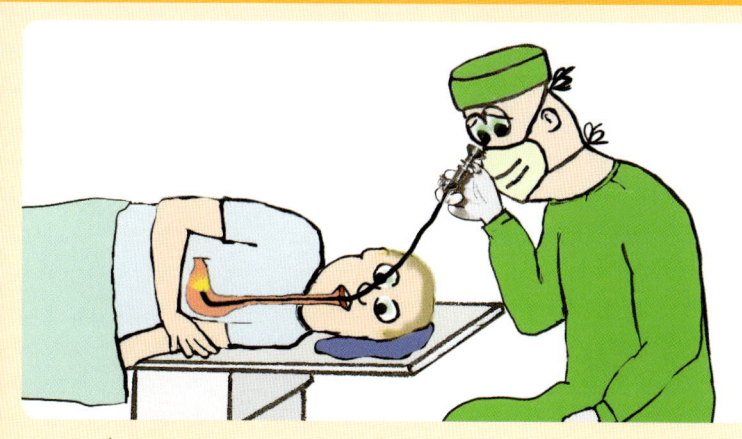

gastroscopy
Magenspiegelung
فیلمبرداری معده

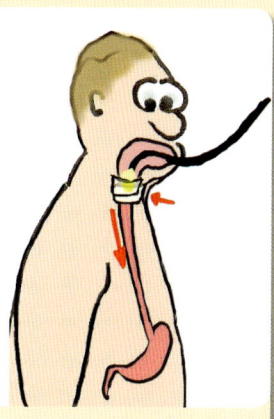

swallow! swallow!
schlucken! schlucken!
قورت بدهید! قورت بدهید!

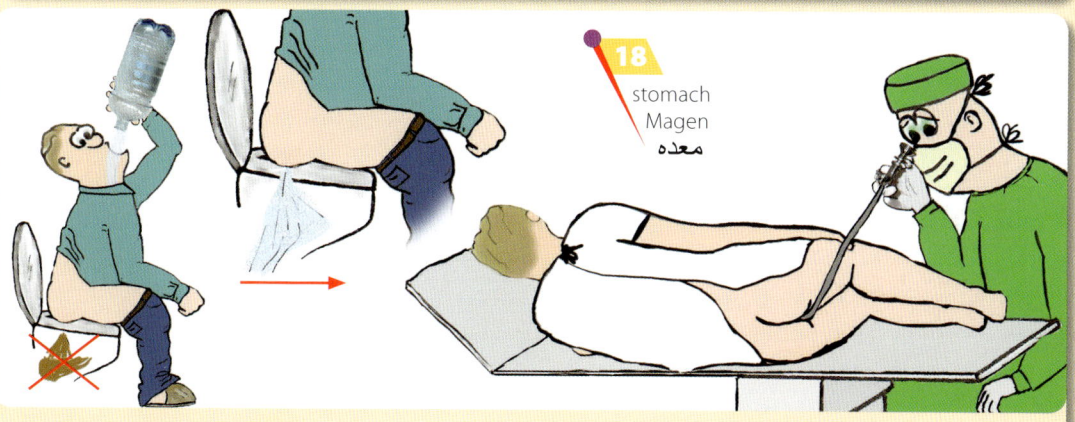

18 stomach / Magen / معده

empty the bowels before – like water
vorher abführen – wie Wasser
یبوست را برطرف کنید - مثل آب

colonoscopy
Darmspiegelung
معاینه روده با دوربین

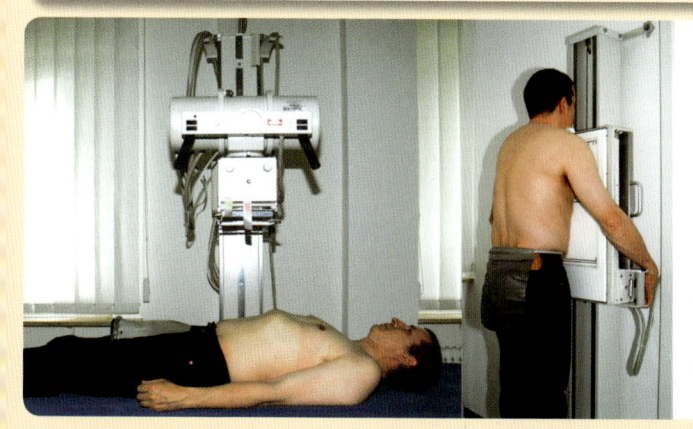

x-raying
Röntgen
عکس رادیولوژی

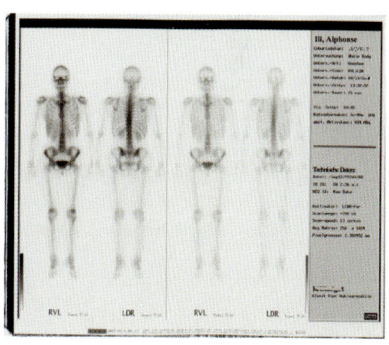

skeletal scintigraphy
Skelettszintigraphie
عکسبرداری استخوان

Examination
At the x-raying

Untersuchung
Beim Röntgen

معاینه
موقع عکس رادیولوژی

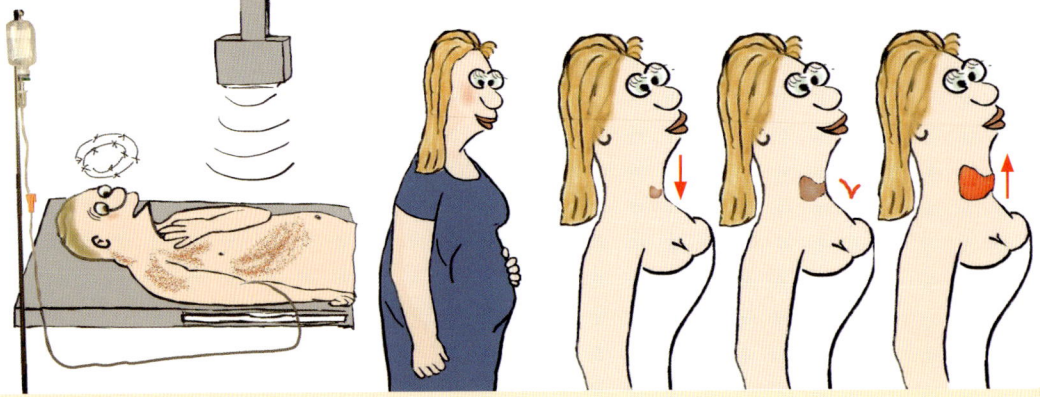

allergy to contrast media
Kontrastmittelallergie
حساسیت به رادیولوژی

pregnant?
schwanger?
حامله؟

thyroid gland
Schilddrüse
غده تیروئید

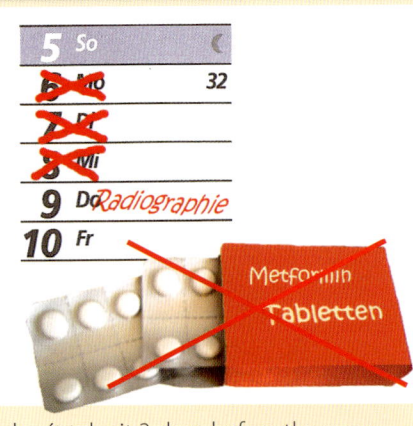

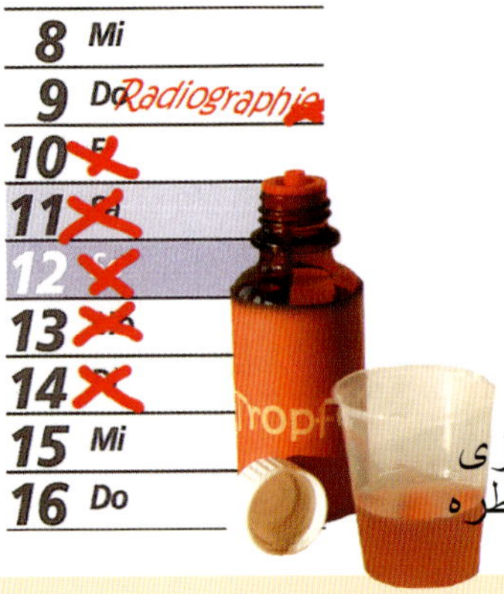

- 40 drops now
  20 drops tonight
  5 days 3 x 20 drops
- sofort 40 Tropfen
  abds. 20 Tropfen
  5 Tage 3 x 20 Tropfen
- فوراً ٤٠ قطره
  شبها ٢٠ قطره
  ٥ روز پشت سرهم روزی
  ٣ دفعه، هر دفعه ٢٠ قطره
- e. g./z. B. Irenat®
  مثلا

don´t take it 3 days before the x-ray
3 Tage vor dem Röntgen nicht einnehmen
٣ روز قبل از رادیولوژی دارو نخورید.

take it after the x-ray
nach dem Röntgen einnehmen
بعد از رادیولوژی دارو بخورید.

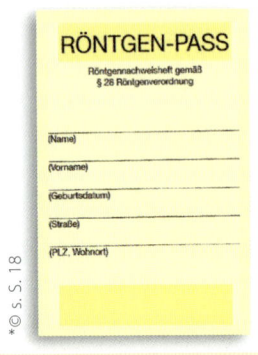

x-ray card
Röntgenpass
دفترچه رادیولوژی

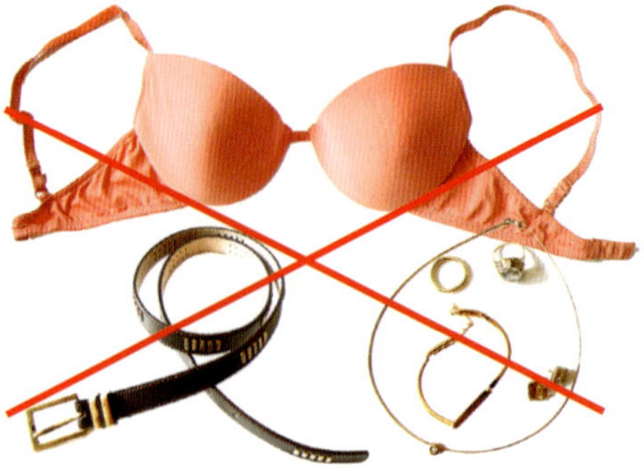

no jewellery/bra/metal
kein Schmuck/BH/Metall
بدون زیورآلات / سینه بند / فلز

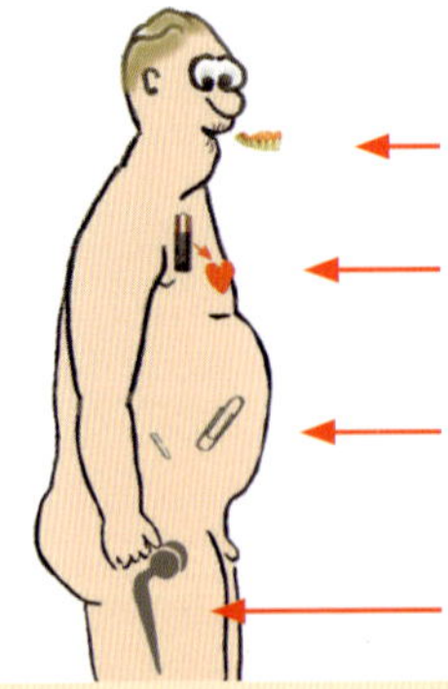

implants/prothesis/pace maker?
Implantate/Prothesen/Schrittmacher?
اندام مصنوعی/پروتز/قلب مصنوعی؟

Examination
At the x-raying

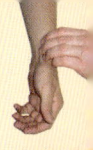

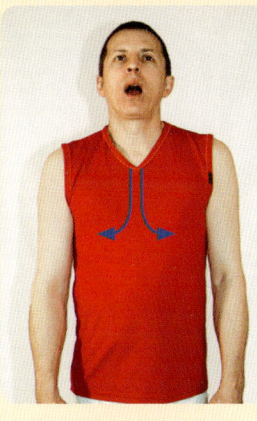

Untersuchung
Beim Röntgen

معاینه
موقع عکس رادیولوژی

take a deep breath
tief einatmen
نفس عمیق بکشید.

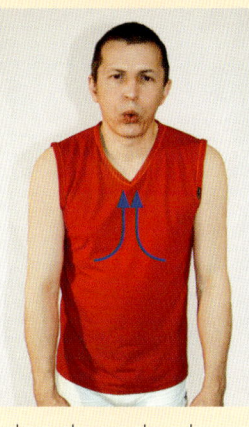

breath out deeply
tief ausatmen
نفس را بیرون دهید.

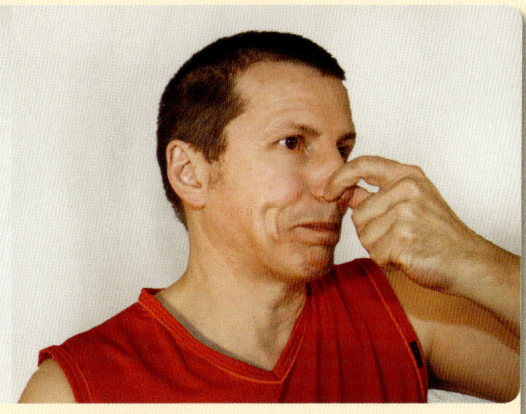

stop breathing
nicht atmen
نفس نکشید.

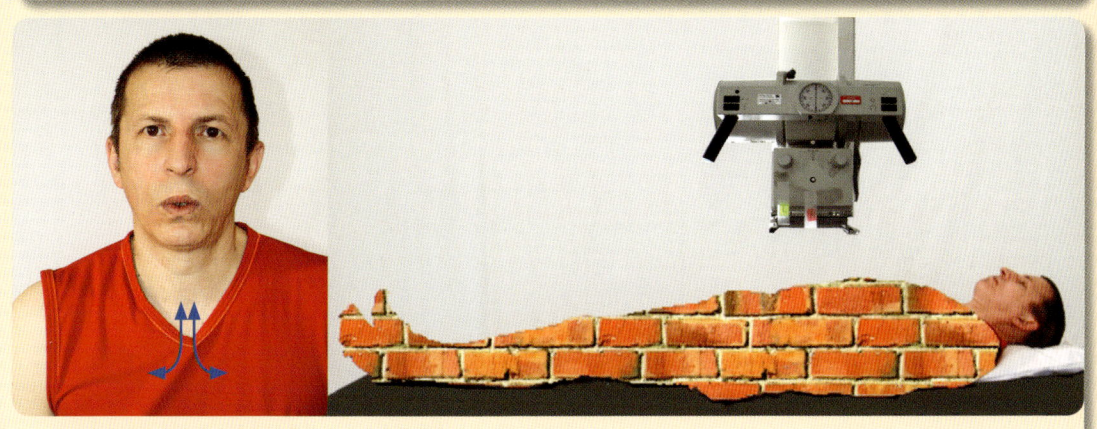

carry on breathing
weiteratmen
به نفس کشیدن ادامه دهید.

don´t move
nicht bewegen
حرکت نکنید.

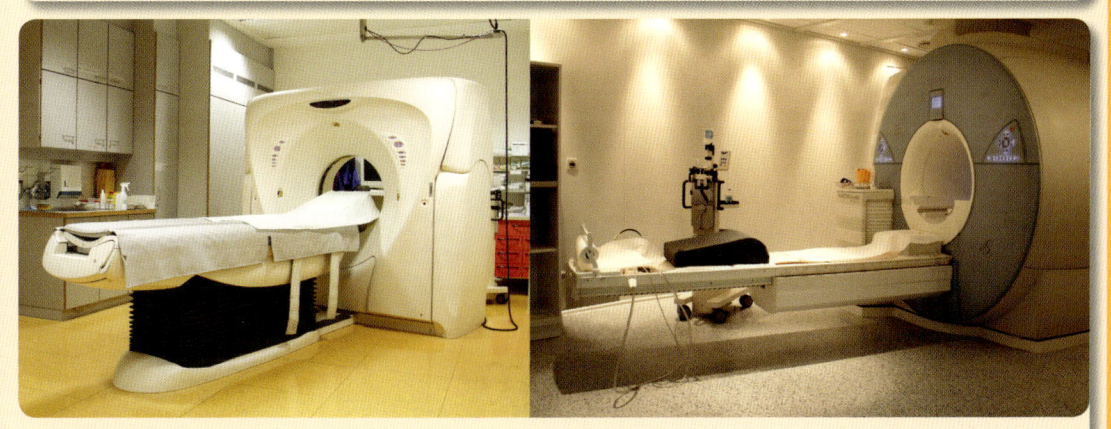

computer-tomography
Computertomographie/CT
توموگرافی

nuclear magnetic resonance
Kernspintomographie/NMR/MRT
توموگرافی هسته ای / ان ام ار / ام ارت

53

| Treatment | Behandlung | درمان |

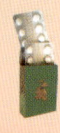

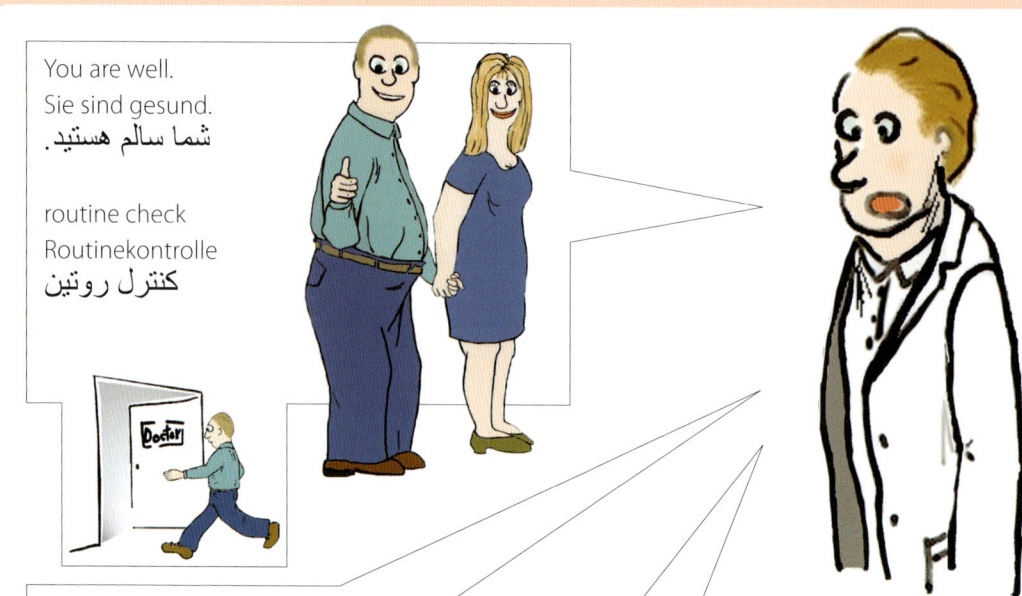

You are well.
Sie sind gesund.
شما سالم هستید.

routine check
Routinekontrolle
کنترل روتین

no treatment
keine Behandlung
بدون درمان

check up only
nur Kontrolle
فقط کنترل

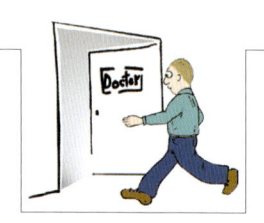

not serious
nicht gefährlich
خطرناک نیست.

serious illness
ernste Erkrankung
بیماری جدی

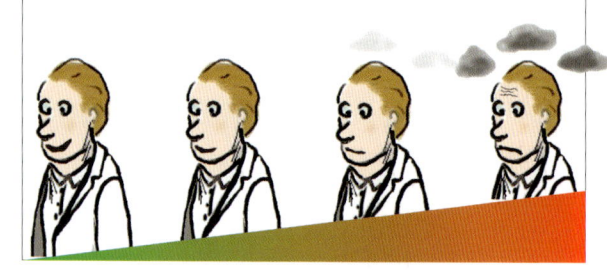

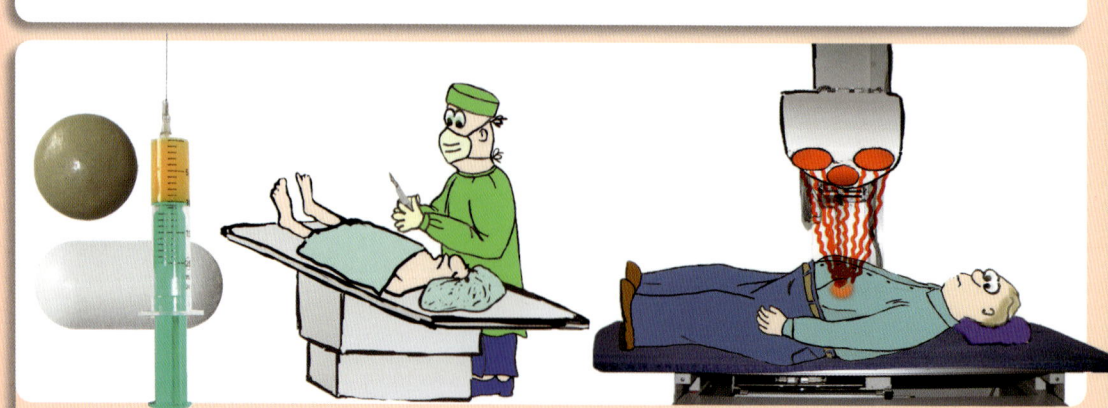

medicine
Medikamente
دارو

operation
Operation
عمل جراحی

irradiation
Bestrahlung
اشعه

Treatment — Behandlung — درمان

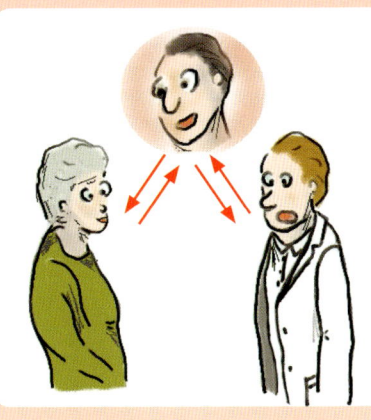

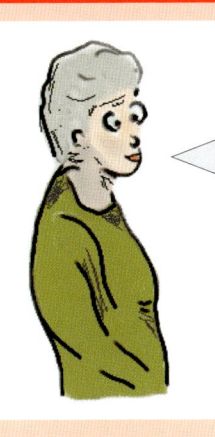

Please write down the name of the disease.

لطفا بیماری خود را برای من بنویسید.

Schreiben Sie mir bitte den Namen der Krankheit auf.

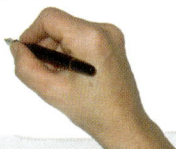

interpreter
Dolmetscher
مترجم

name of the disease
Name der Krankheit
نام بیماری

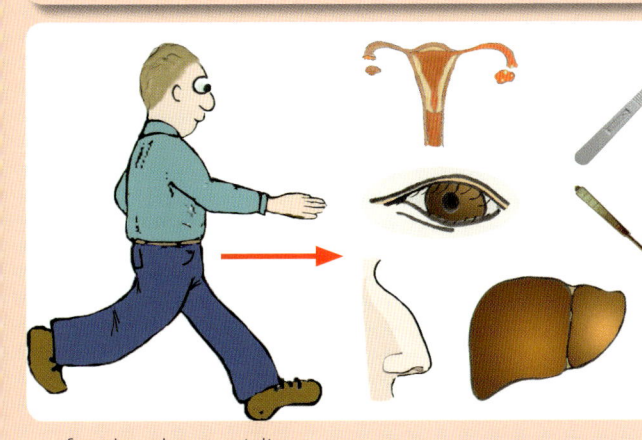

Schmerztherapie
Hautarzt
Psychotherapie

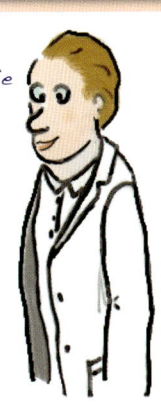

referral to the specialist
zum Facharzt gehen
پهلوی دکتر متخصص بروید.

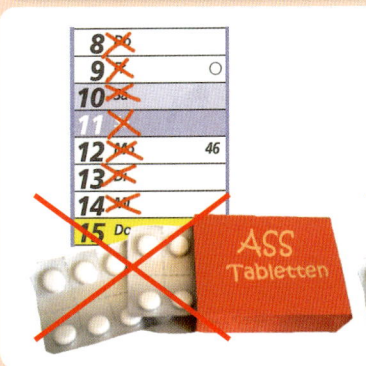

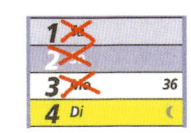

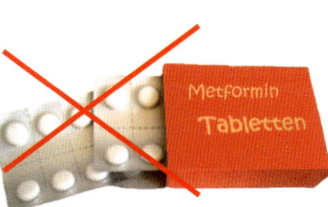

7 days before no ASS (Aspirin®)
7 Tage vorher kein ASS
۷ روز قبل آسپیرین نخورید.

3 days before no metformine
3 Tage vorher kein Metformin
۳ روز قبل متفورمین نخورید.

make a report
Protokoll führen
صورتجلسه بنویسید.

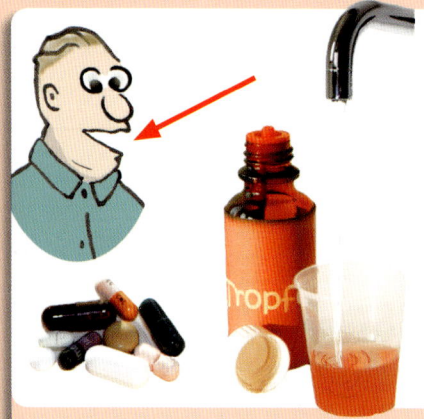

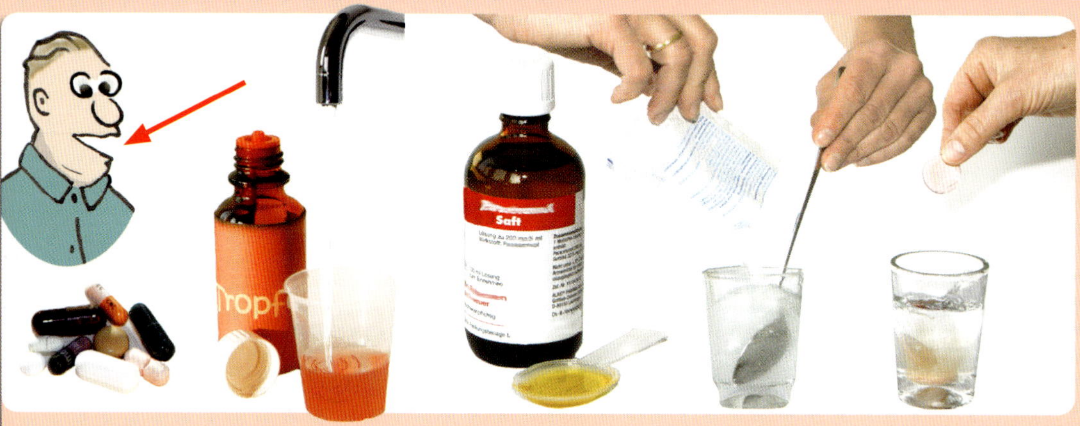

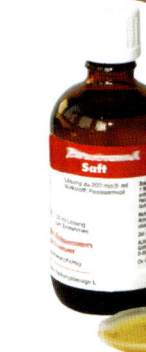

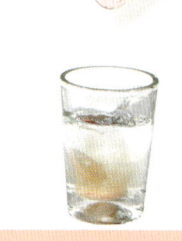

Treatment	Behandlung	درمان
Medicine	Medikamente	داروها

tablets	drops	dilution	measuring spoon	powder	effervescent tablet
Tabletten	Tropfen	Saft	Messlöffel	Pulver	Brausetablette
قرصها	قطره ها	آب میوه	قاشق اندازه گیری	پودر	قرص جوشان

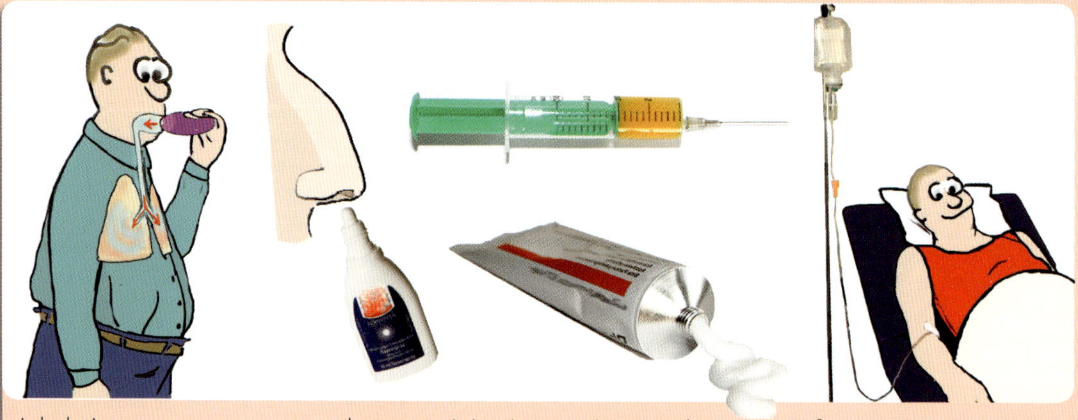

inhalation	nasal spray	injection	ointment/cream	infusion
Inhalation	Nasenspray	Spritze	Creme/Salbe	Infusion/Tropf
نفس عمیق کشیدن	اسپری دماغ	آمپول	کرم/پماد	تزریق سرم

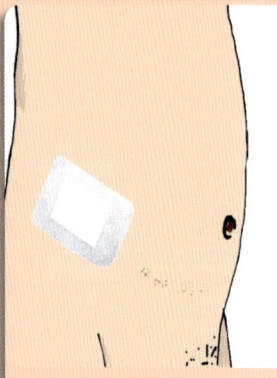

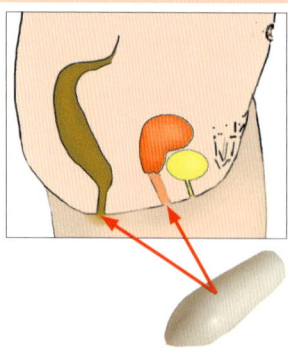

bandage/patch	suppository	hip bath	foot bath
Pflaster	Zäpfchen	Sitzbad	Fußbad
چسب زخم	شیاف	حمام نشسته	حمام پا

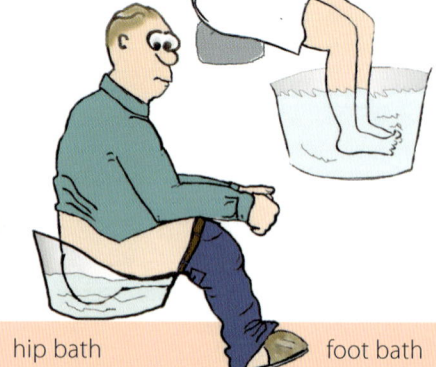

Treatment	Behandlung	درمان
Application	Medikamenteneinnahme	خوردن داروها

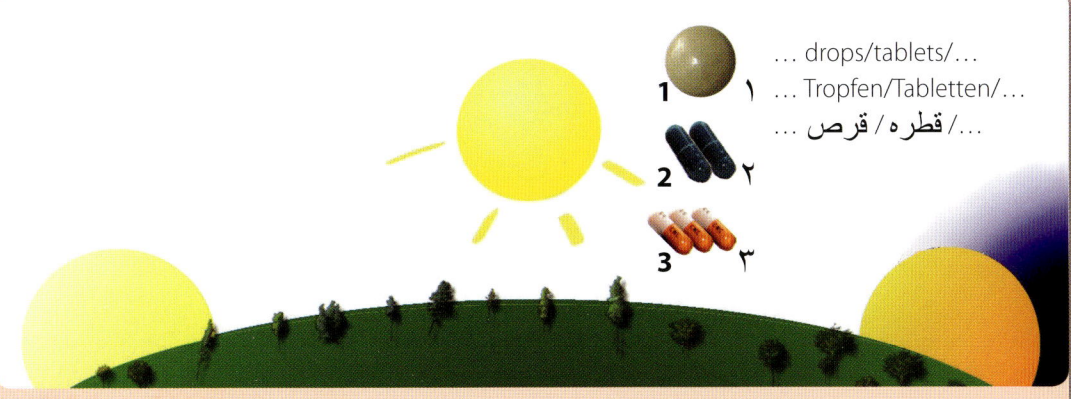

... drops/tablets/...
... Tropfen/Tabletten/...
... قرص / قطره /...

in the morning	at noon	in the evening	at night
morgens	mittags	abends	zur Nacht
صبح	ظهر	عصر	شب

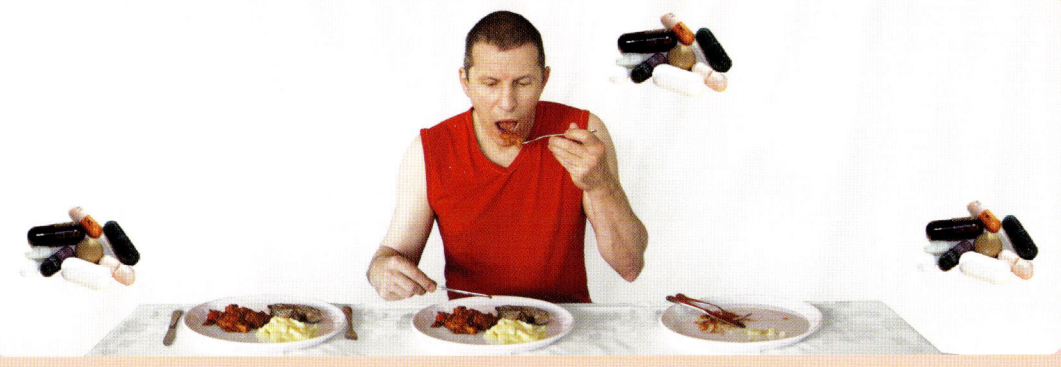

before	during	after the meals
vor	zum	nach dem Essen
قبل	هنگام	بعد از غذا

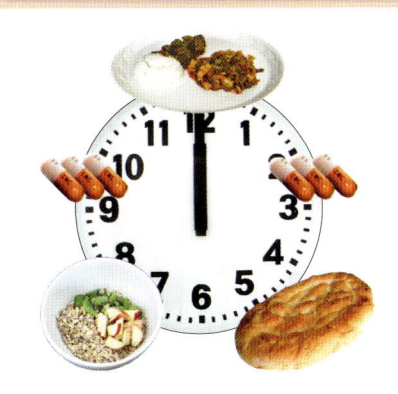

between the meals
zwischen den Mahlzeit
بین وعده های غذائی

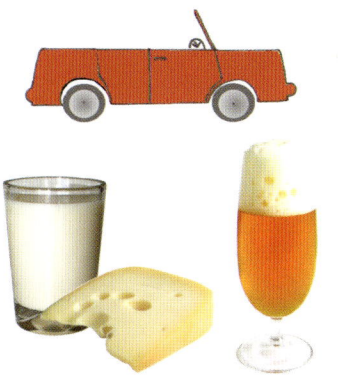

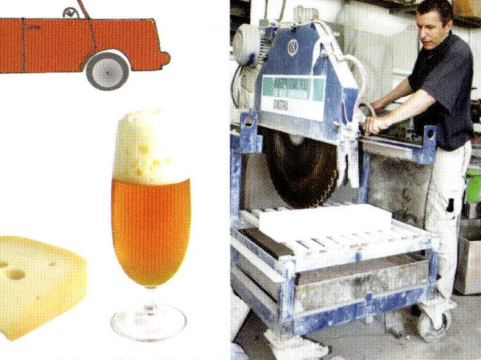

don't take concurrently ...
Medikament nicht zusammen mit ...
دارو را با ... مصرف نکنید.

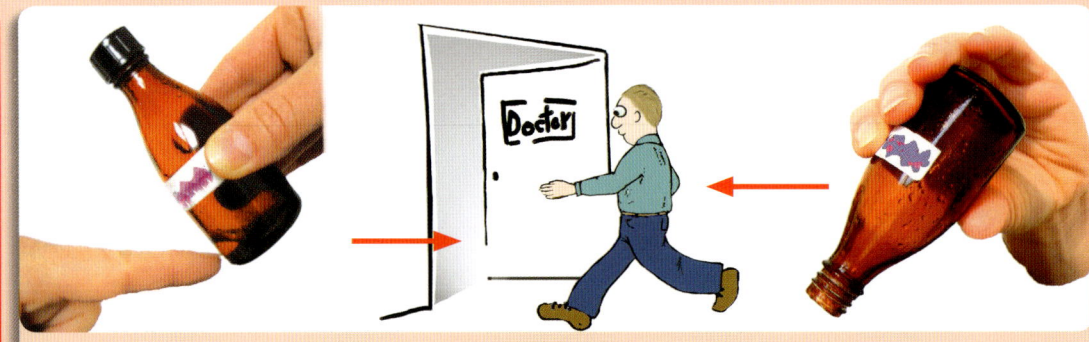

Treatment	Behandlung	درمان
Application	Medikamenteneinnahme	خوردن داروها

before the medicine is finished
bevor die Medizin alle ist
قبل از اینکه دارو تمام شود.

another appointment
Wiederkommen
برگشتن

when the medicine is finished
wenn die Medizin alle ist
وقتی که دارو تمام شده.

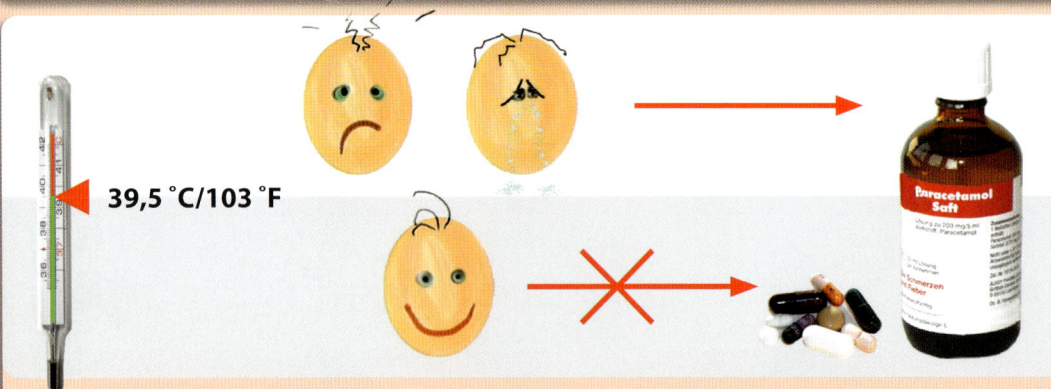

39,5 °C/103 °F

additional: when fever   when pain   if required
zusätzlich: bei Fieber   bei Schmerzen   bei Bedarf
              با تب   با درد   هنگام نیاز   اضافی :

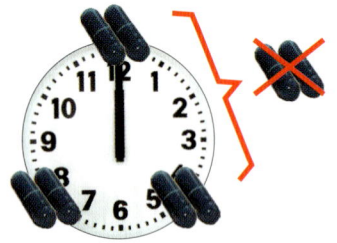

*4 hours   Stunden   * ٤ ساعت
... hours Stunden   ... ساعت
... tablets Tabletten ... قرصها
... drops Tropfen   ... قطره ها

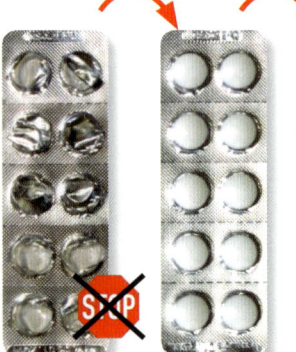

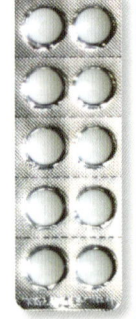

not more/no more often than every ...*   ingest until the medicine is finished
nicht mehr/nicht öfter als alle ...*
                                          don´t discontinue the administration
              einnehmen bis die Tabletten alle sind   Tabletten nicht unterbrechen

بیشتر نه/ بیشتر از هر ... ساعت نه
خوردن قرصها را قطع نکنید.   قرصها بخورید تا وقتی که تمام شوند.

Treatment
Attitude/applications

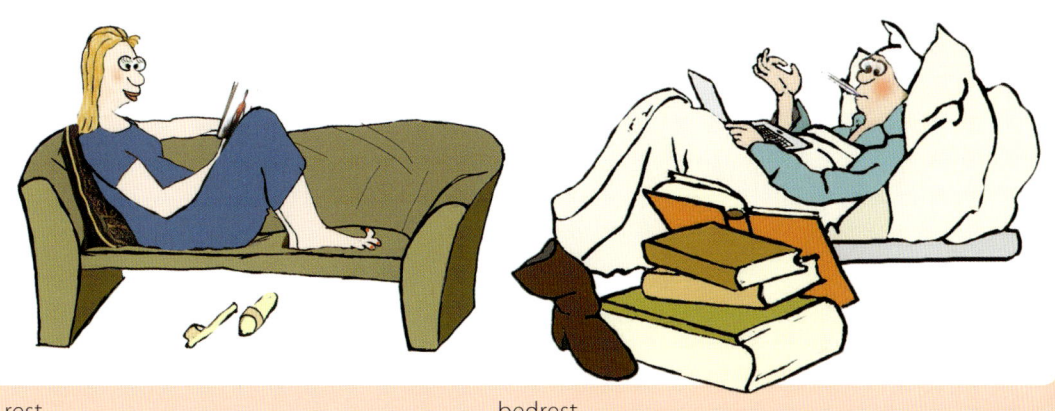

Behandlung
Verhalten/Anwendungen

درمان
رفتار / استفاده

rest
Schonung
مراقبت

bedrest
Bettruhe
استراحت

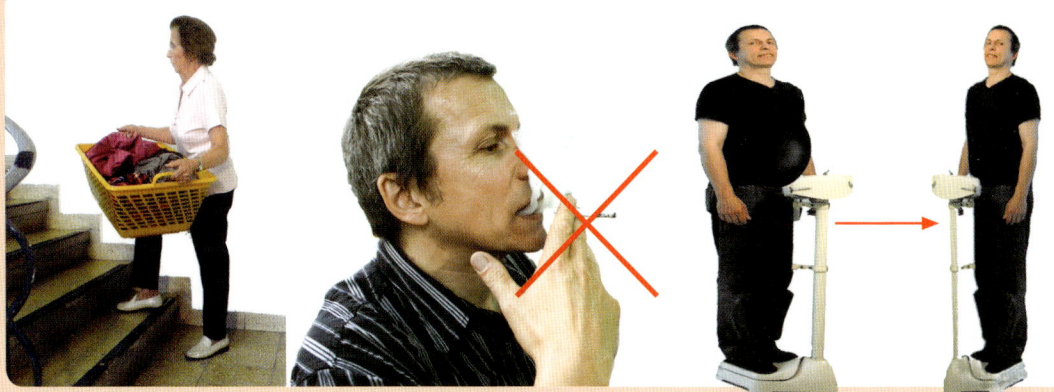

lifting – ... kg – don´t lift
heben – ... kg – nicht heben
بلند کردن -... کیلو - بلند نکنید.

don´t smoke
nicht rauchen
سیگار نکشید.

lose weight
Gewicht abnehmen
وزن کم کنید.

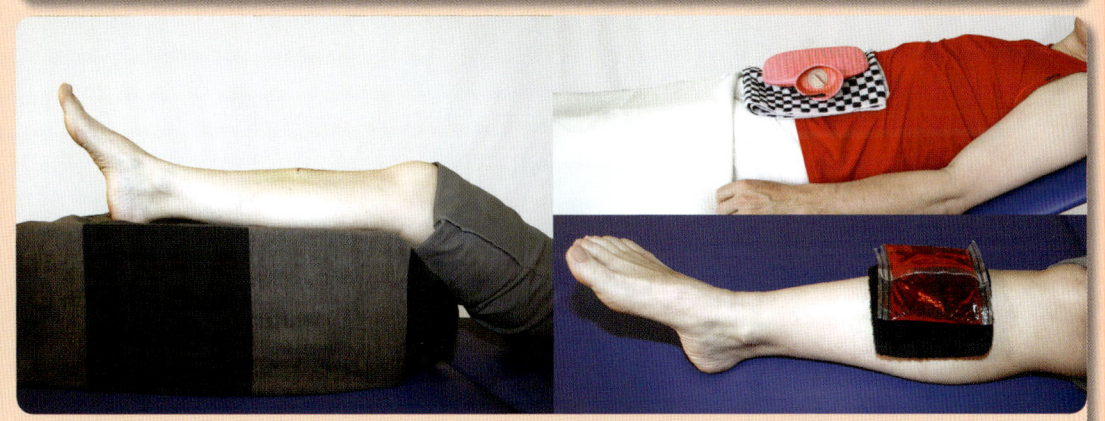

put it up
hochlagern
بالا گذاشتن

warmth
Wärme
گرم نگه داشتن

cooling
kühlen
سرد نگه داشتن

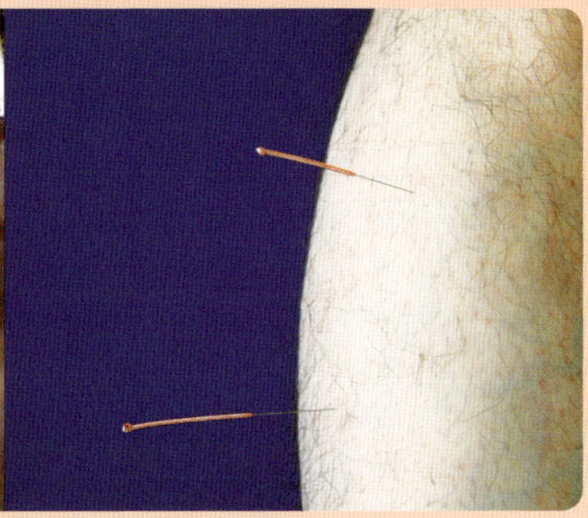

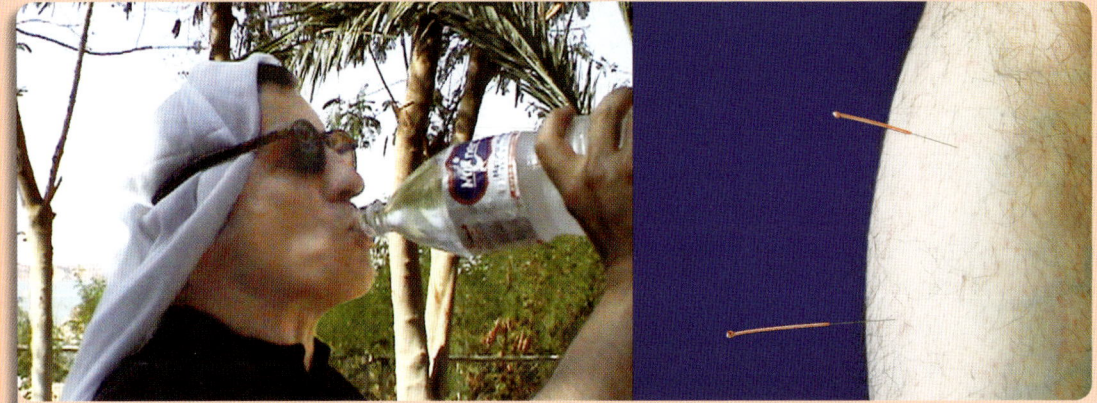

| Treatment | Behandlung | درمان |
| Attitude/applications | Verhalten/Anwendungen | رفتار / استفاده |

shade	cover	sun-glasses	water	acupuncture
Schatten	Kopfschutz	Sonnenbrille	Wasser	Akupunktur
سایه	سر بند	عینک آفتابی	آب	طب سوزنی

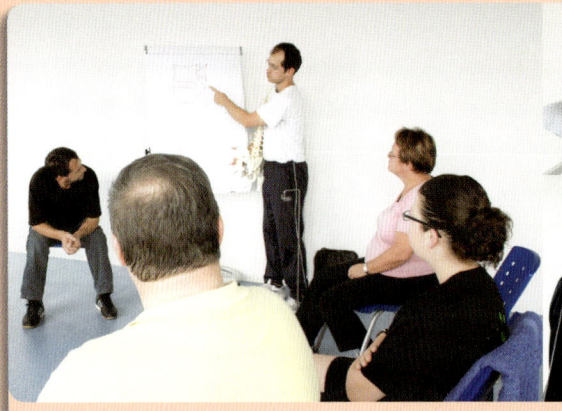

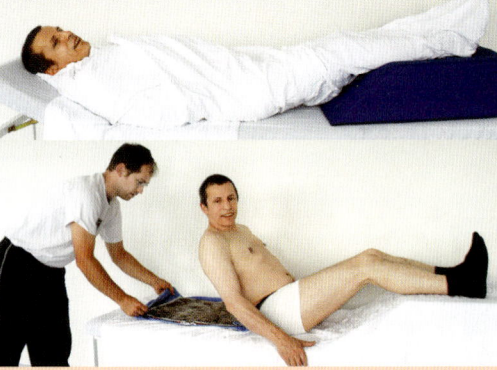

posture training　　　　　　　　fango/mud pack therapy
Rückenschule　　　　　　　　　Fango/Naturmoor
مدرسه کمردرد　　　　　　　　ماساژ با لجن / ماساژ با جلبک

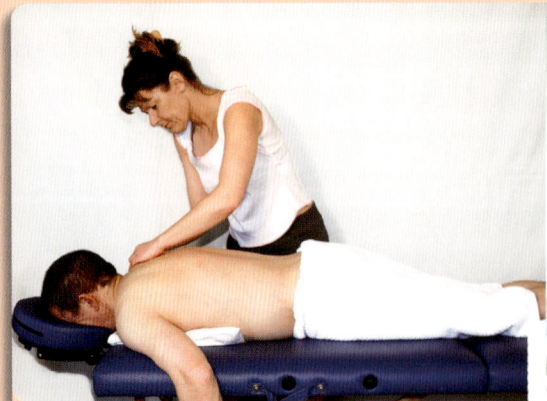

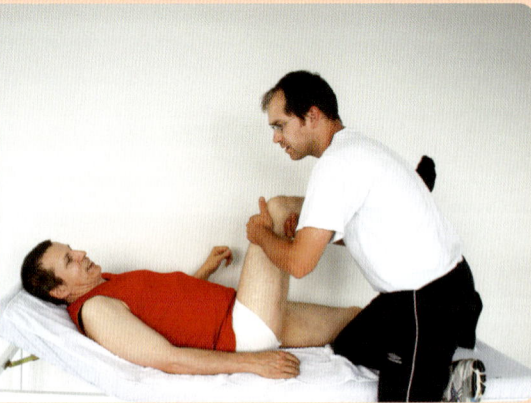

60

massage　　　　　　　　　　manual therapy
Massage　　　　　　　　　　manuelle Therapie
ماساژ　　　　　　　　　　　درمان بوسیله دست

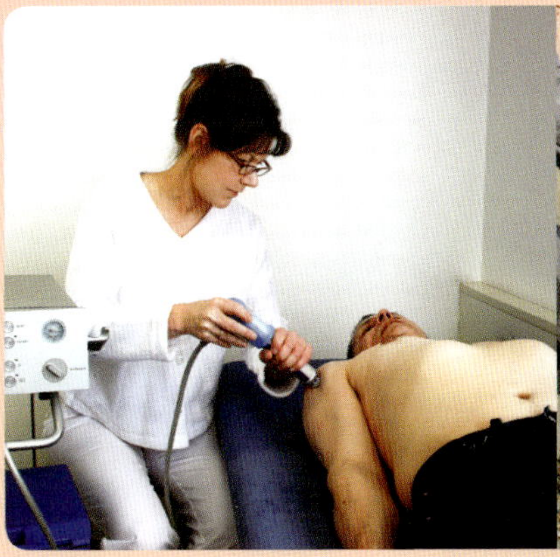

Treatment
Attitude/applications

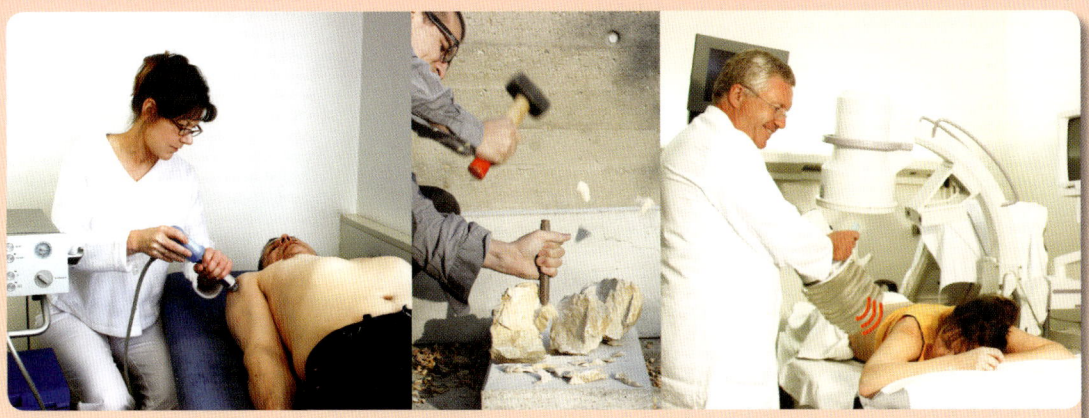

Behandlung
Verhalten/Anwendungen

درمان
رفتار / استفاده

joints	shockwave therapy	kidney
Gelenke	Stoßwellentherapie	Niere
مفاصل	درمان بوسیله ضربه موجی	کلیه

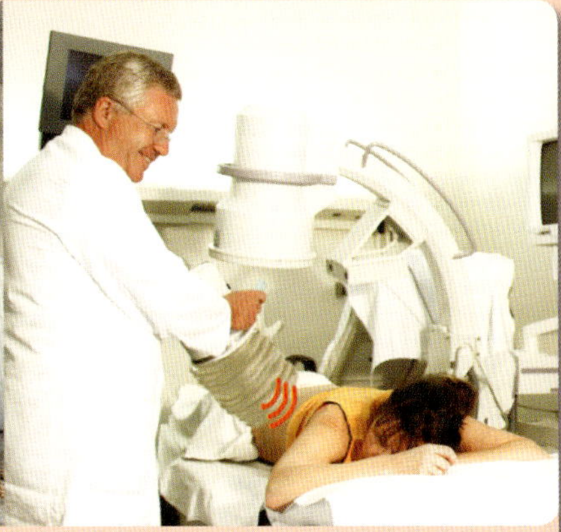

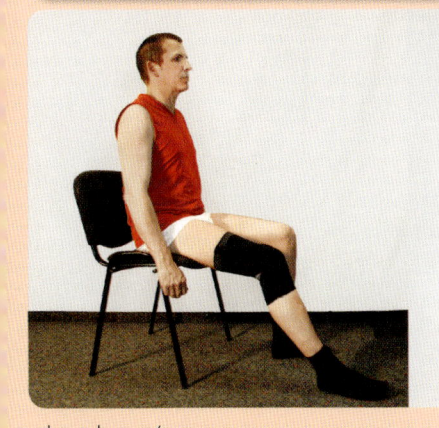

bandages/tapes		booster cushion
Bandagen		Sitzerhöhung
پانسمان		بالا بردن صندلی

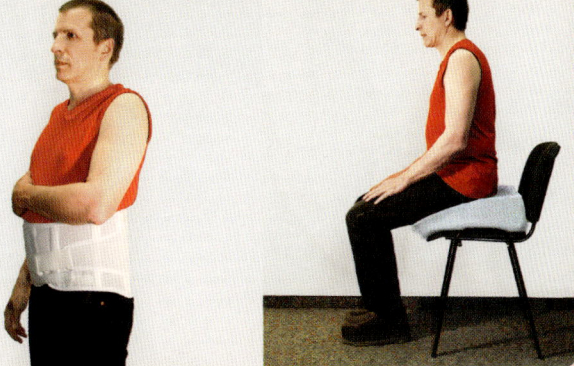

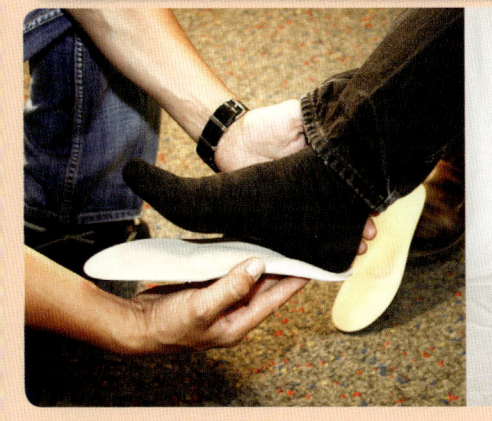

insole	surgical hose	
Einlegesohlen	Kompressionsstrümpfe/Gummistrümpfe	
لائی کف پا	جوراب کشی / جوراب لاستیکی	

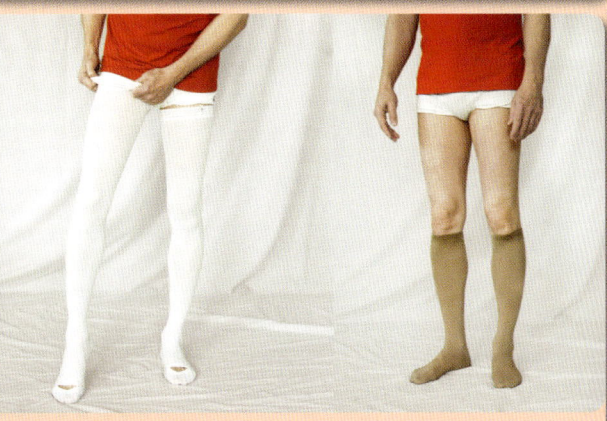

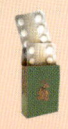

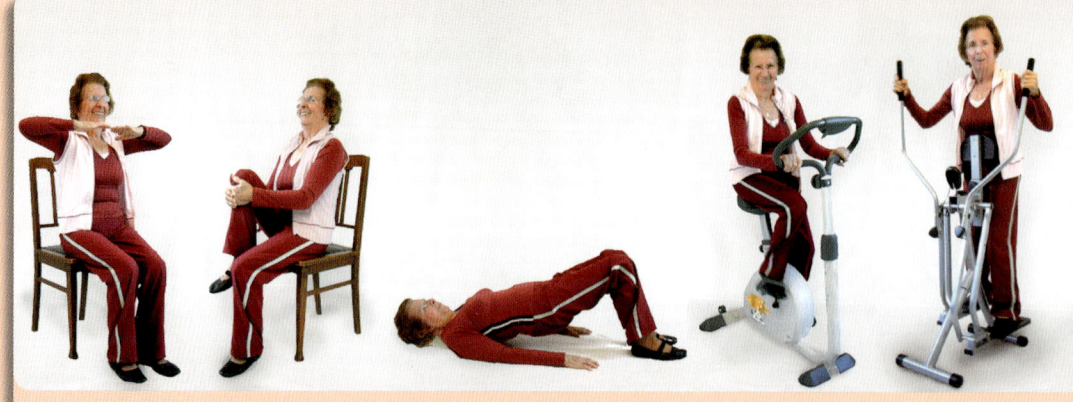

Treatment	Behandlung	درمان
Attitude/applications	Verhalten/Anwendungen	رفتار / استفاده

gymnastics
Gymnastik
ژیمناستیک

pelvic floor gymnastic
Beckenbodengymnastik
ژیمناستیک درازکش

exercise with training equipments
Trainieren mit Geräten
تمرین با ماشینهای بدنسازی

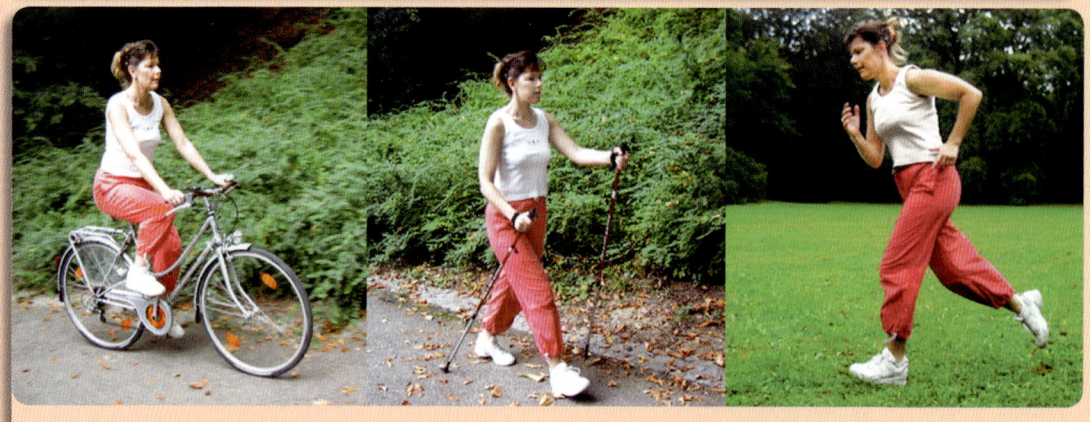

cycling
Fahrrad fahren
دوچرخه سواری

walking
Walken
پیاده روی

jogging
Joggen
دویدن

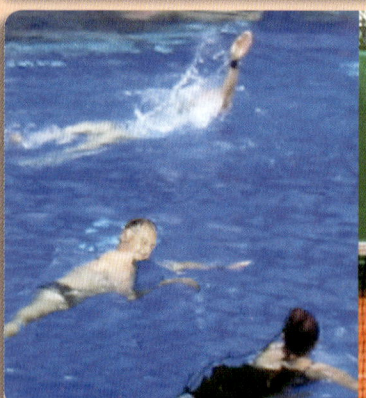

swimming
Schwimmen
شنا

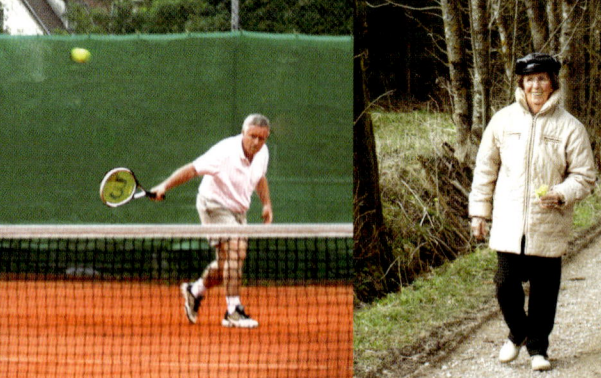

tennis
Tennis
تنیس

motor activity/ambulate
Bewegung/Gehen
حرکت / راه رفتن

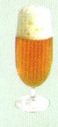

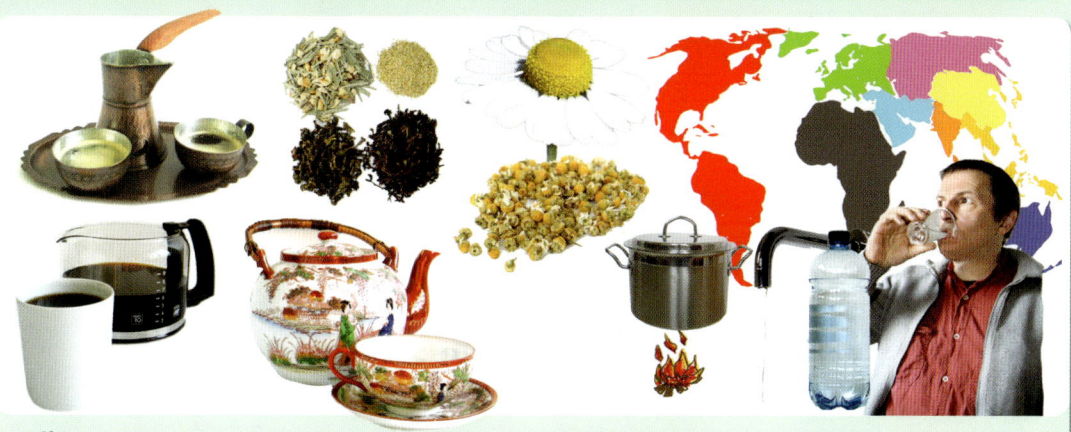

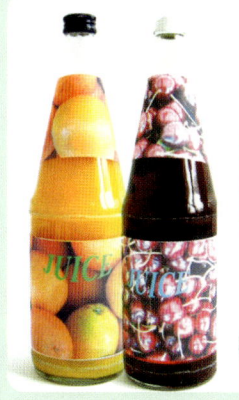

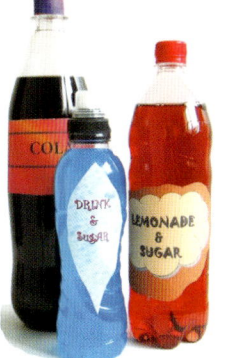

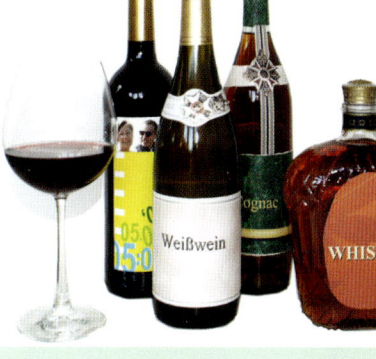

| Nutrition | Ernährung | تغذیه |

coffee	tea	water	Where drunk?	boiled?
Kaffee	Tee	Wasser	Wo getrunken?	abgekocht?
قهوه	چای	آب	کجا نوشیدید؟	جوشاندید؟

juice	with sugar	red wine – white wine	wodka whisky … beer
Obstsaft	mit Zucker	Rotwein – Weißwein	Wodka Whisky … Bier
آب میوه	با شکر	شراب قرمز - شراب سفید	ودکا ویسکی ... آبجو

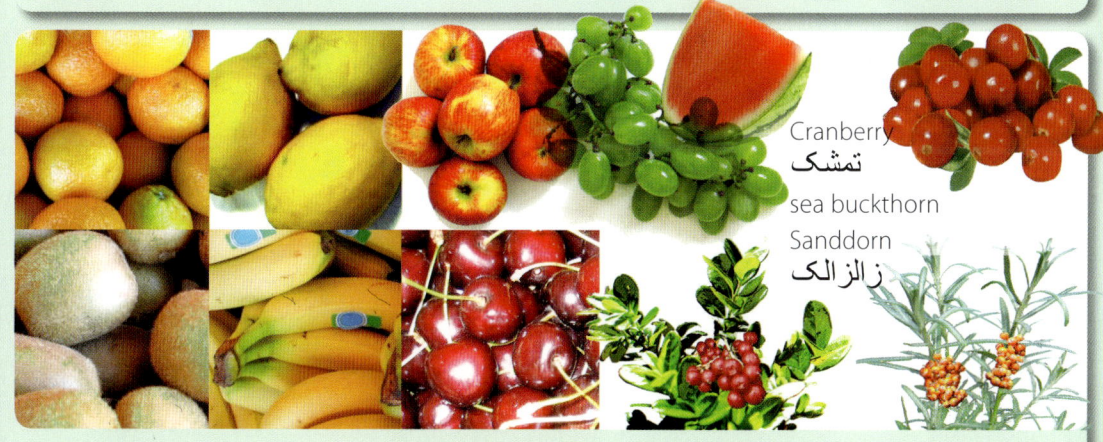

Cranberry
تمشک

sea buckthorn
Sanddorn
زالزالک

fruit: citrus fruits – banane – apple – grapes – melon – red fruits – lingonberry
Obst: Zitrusfrüchte – Bananen – Apfel – Weintrauben – Melone – rotes Obst – Preiselbeere
میوه: مرکبات - موز - سیب - انگور - هندوانه - میوجات قرمز - زالزالک قرمز

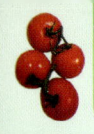

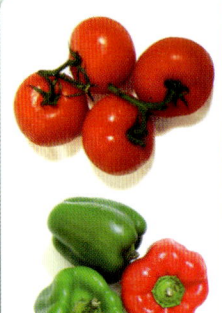

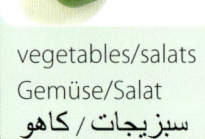

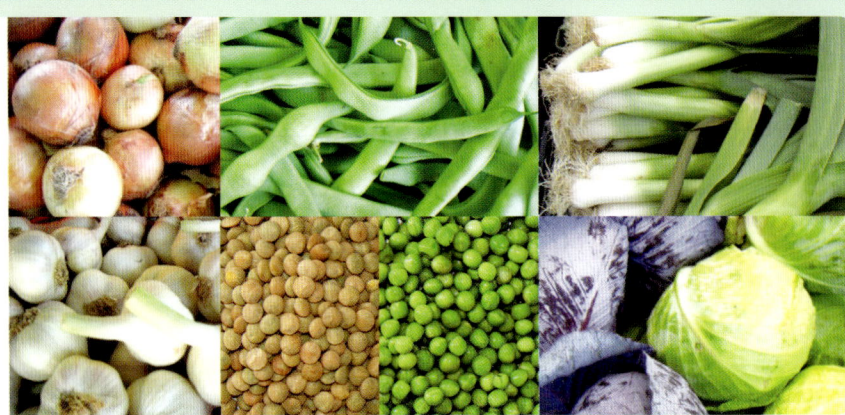

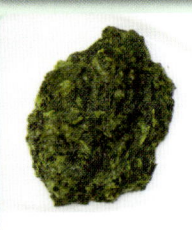

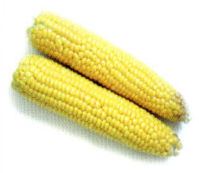

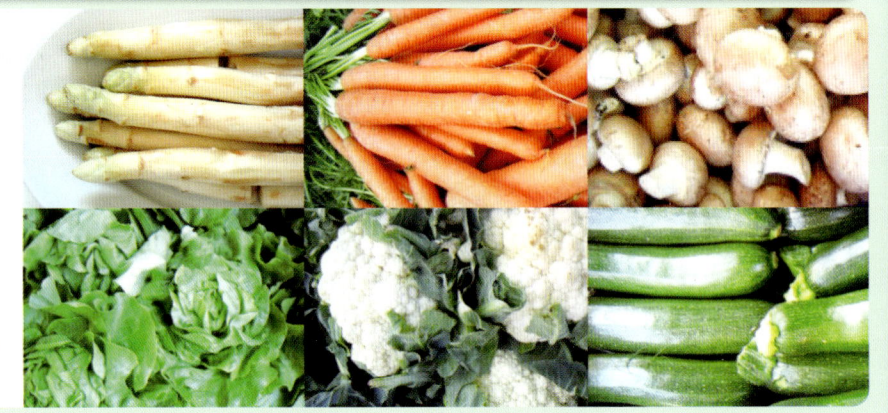

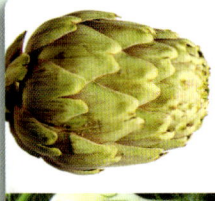

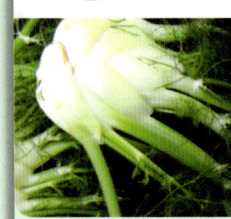

Nutrition	Ernährung	تغذیه

vegetables/salats
Gemüse/Salat
سبزیجات / کاهو

vegetables/salats
Gemüse/Salat
سبزیجات / کاهو

artichoke	fennel	ginger	caraway	hot	fish
Artischocke	Fenchel	Ingwer	Kümmel	Scharfes	Fisch
آرتیشو	رازیانه	زنجبیل	زیره	ادویه تند	ماهی

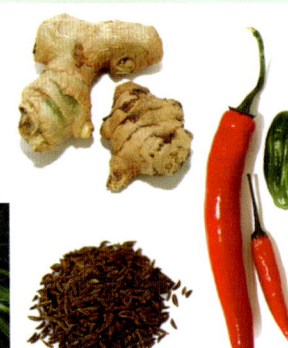

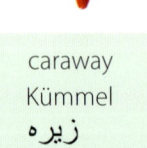

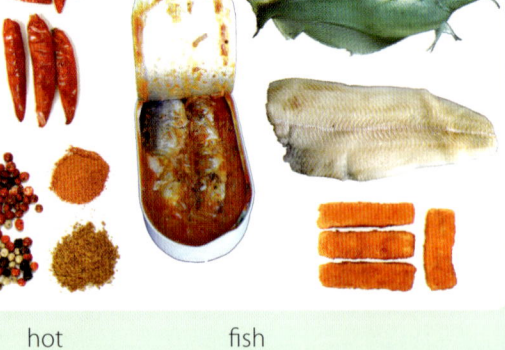

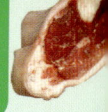

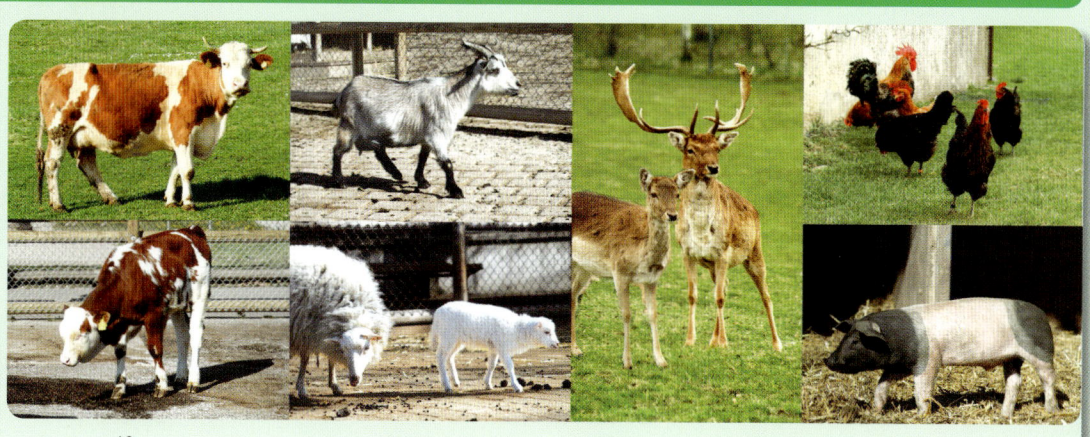

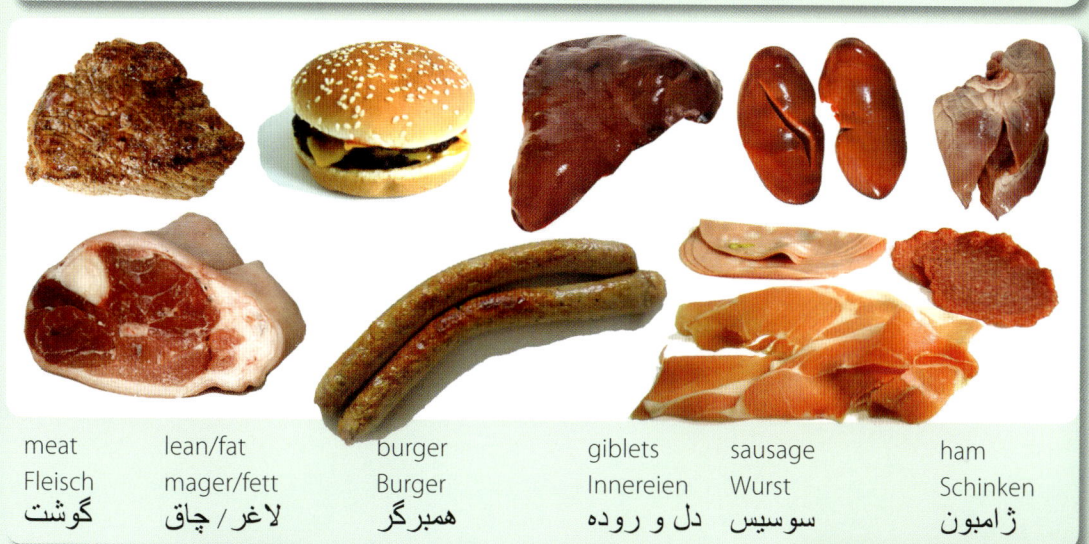

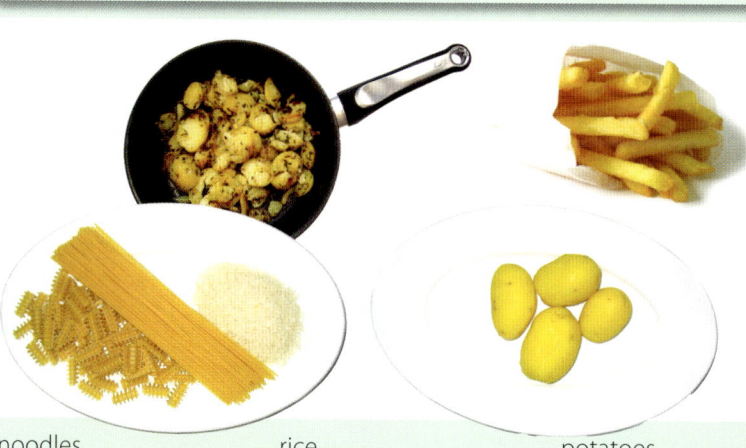

Nutrition   Ernährung   تغذیه

cow – calf	goat sheep – lamb	deer	poultry	pork
Kuh – Kalb	Ziege Schaf – Lamm	Wild	Geflügel	Schwein
گوساله - گاو	بز بره - گوسفند	وحشی	پرنده	خوک

meat	lean/fat	burger	giblets	sausage	ham
Fleisch	mager/fett	Burger	Innereien	Wurst	Schinken
گوشت	لاغر / چاق	همبرگر	دل و روده	سوسیس	ژامبون

noodles	rice	potatoes	french fries
Nudeln	Reis	Kartoffeln	Pommes frites
ماکارونی	برنج	سیب زمینی	سیب زمینی سرخ کرده

65

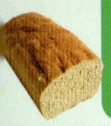

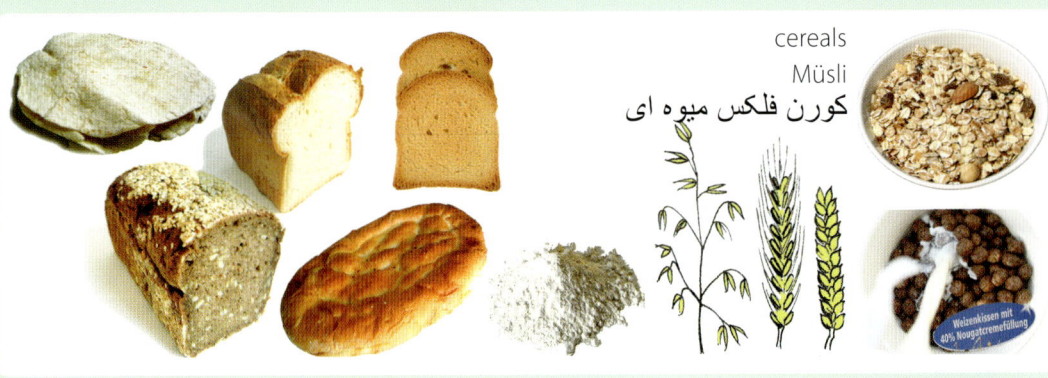

| Nutrition | Ernährung | تغذیه |

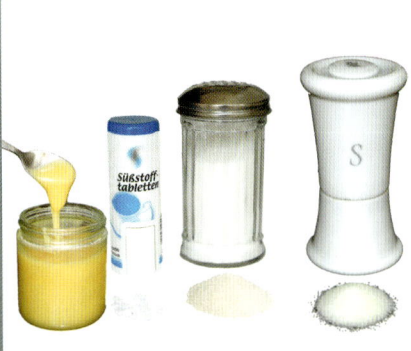

				cereals		
				Müsli		
				کورن فلکس میوه ای		
wholewheat bread	whitebread	Zwieback	wheat	rye	oat	sweet flakes chococrispies
Vollkornbrot	Weißbrot	Zwieback	Weizen	Roggen	Hafer	Schokoflakes
نان سیاه	نان سفید	نان سوخاری	گندم	چاودار	جو	کورن فلکس شکلاتی

flaxseed
Leinsamen
بذر کتان

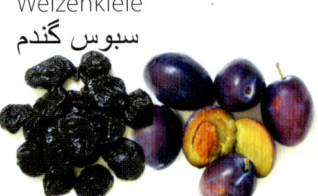

wheat germ
Weizenkleie
سبوس گندم

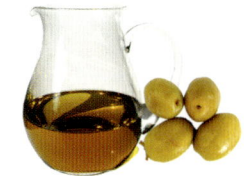

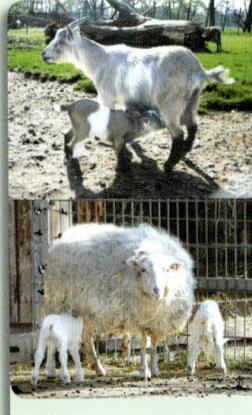

sweeteners	salt	plums/prune	rape oil	olive oil
Süßstoffe	Salz	Back-/Pflaumen	Rapsöl	Olivenöl
قند و شکر	نمک	آلو بخارا	روغن نباتی	روغن زیتون

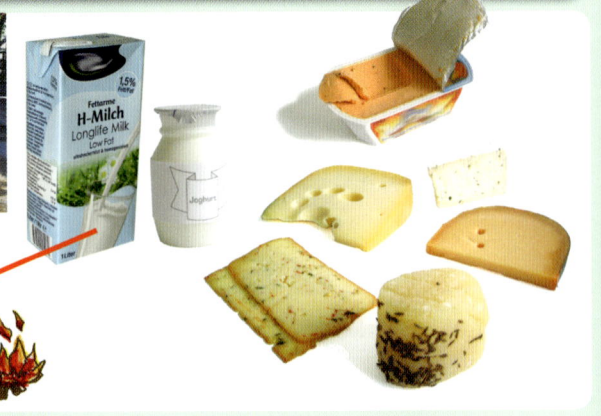

milk	pasteurized/heated	dairy products: e. g. cheese – yoghurt
Milch	pasteurisiert/erhitzt	Milchprodukte: z. B. Käse – Joghurt
شیر	پاستوریزه - گرم	لبنیات: مثل پنیر - ماست

| Nutrition | Ernährung | تغذیه |

eggs	pan	cooking pot
Eier	Bratpfanne	Kochtopf
تخم مرغ	ماهی تابه	قابلمه

nuts	flips	chips	cake	chocolate	sweets
Nüsse	Flips	Chips	Kuchen	Schokolade	Süßigkeiten
بادام زمینی	پفک	چیپس	کیک	شکلات	شیرینیجات

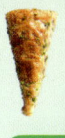

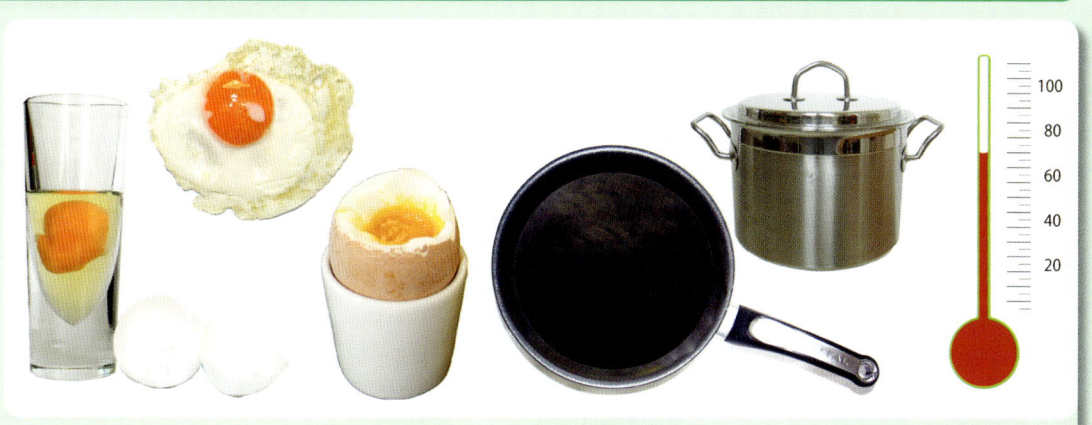

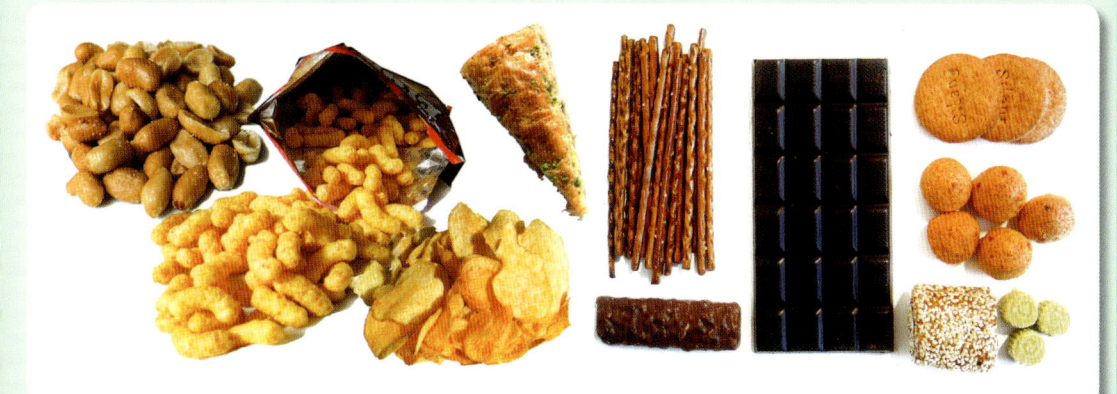

BE-TABELLE

Nährmittel	1 BE
Kartoffeln	
Kartoffeln	80 g
Kartoffelbrei	100 g
Pommes Frites	35 g
Hülsenfrüchte	90 g
Rote Beete	140 g
Brot	
Brötchen	25 g
Toast	25 g
Weizenmischbrot	25 g
Vollkornbrot	30 g
Milch und Milchprodukte	
Vollmilch 3,5%	¼ l
Obst	
Ananas	90 g
Apfel	100 g
Apfelsine	180 g
Erdbeeren	200 g
Himbeeren	200 g
Honigmelone	130 g
Kirschen	110 g
Kiwi	120 g
Wassermelone	250 g
Weintrauben	80 g

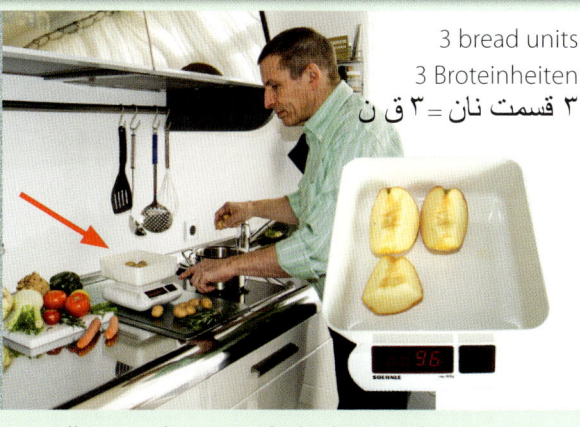

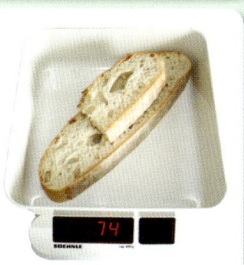

3 bread units
3 Broteinheiten
۳ قسمت نان = ۳ ق ن

1 bread unit
1 Broteinheit = 1 BE
۱ قسمت نان = ۱ ق ن

diabetics: weigh food partially according to carbohydrate exchange-scale
Diabetiker: Essen z. T. abwiegen nach Broteinheiten-Tabelle
کسانی که دیابت دارند: غذا را تا اندازه ای بوسیله جدول قسمت نان وزن کنید.

At the hospital
Where do I find ...?

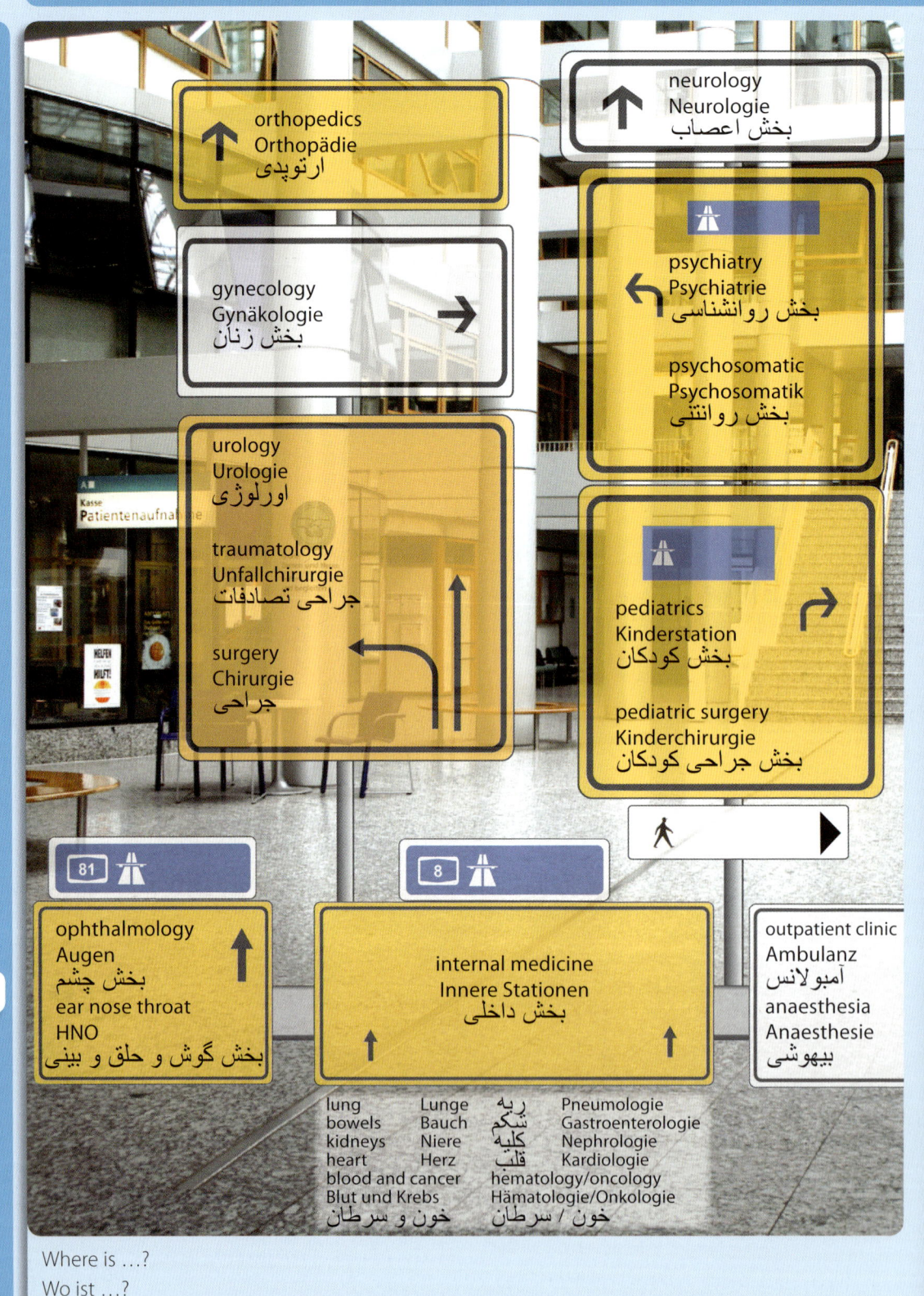

Im Krankenhaus
Wo finde ich ...?

در بیمارستان
... کجاست؟

orthopedics
Orthopädie
ارتوپدی

neurology
Neurologie
بخش اعصاب

gynecology
Gynäkologie
بخش زنان

psychiatry
Psychiatrie
بخش روانشناسی

psychosomatic
Psychosomatik
بخش روانتنی

urology
Urologie
اورلوژی

traumatology
Unfallchirurgie
جراحی تصادفات

surgery
Chirurgie
جراحی

pediatrics
Kinderstation
بخش کودکان

pediatric surgery
Kinderchirurgie
بخش جراحی کودکان

ophthalmology
Augen
بخش چشم
ear nose throat
HNO
بخش گوش و حلق و بینی

internal medicine
Innere Stationen
بخش داخلی

outpatient clinic
Ambulanz
آمبولانس
anaesthesia
Anaesthesie
بیهوشی

lung	Lunge	ریه	Pneumologie
bowels	Bauch	شکم	Gastroenterologie
kidneys	Niere	کلیه	Nephrologie
heart	Herz	قلب	Kardiologie
blood and cancer	Blut und Krebs	خون / سرطان	Hämatologie/Onkologie
		خون و سرطان	hematology/oncology

Where is ...?
Wo ist ...?
... کجاست؟

At the hospital
About the procedure

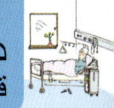

Im Krankenhaus
Zum Eingriff

در بیمارستان
قبل از عمل جراحی

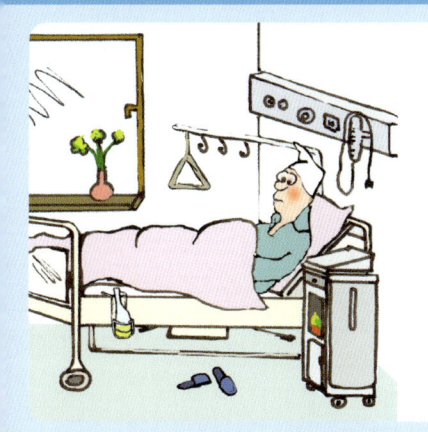

inpatient	outpatient	local anaesthesia
stationär	ambulant	örtliche Betäubung
عمل جراحی با بستری شدن	عمل جراحی سرپائی	بیحسی موضعی

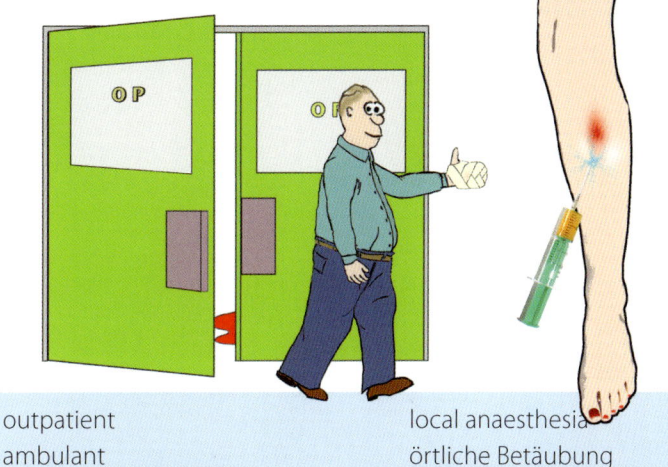

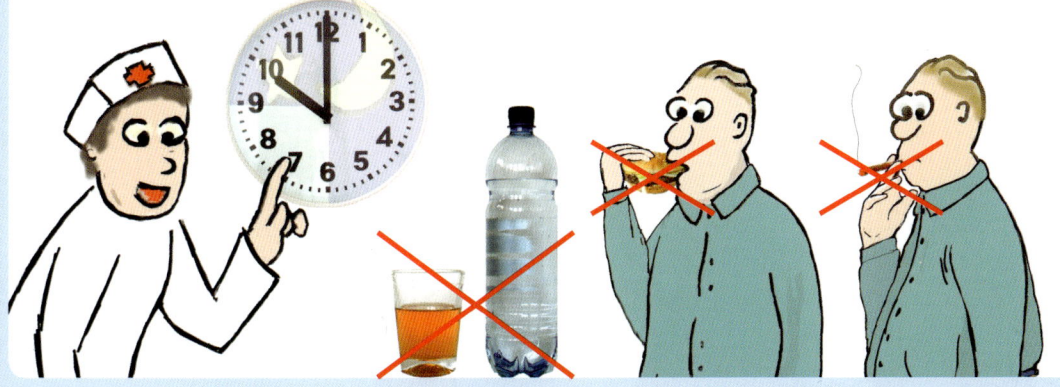

pre-anesthesia discussion	operation: small	medium	large
Narkosevorgespräch	Operation: klein	mittel	groß
آمادگی بیمار برای بیهوشی	کوچک	متوسط	بزرگ — عمل جراحی:

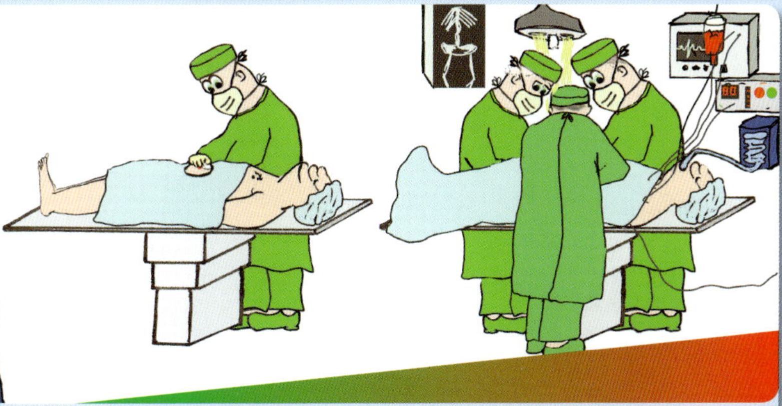

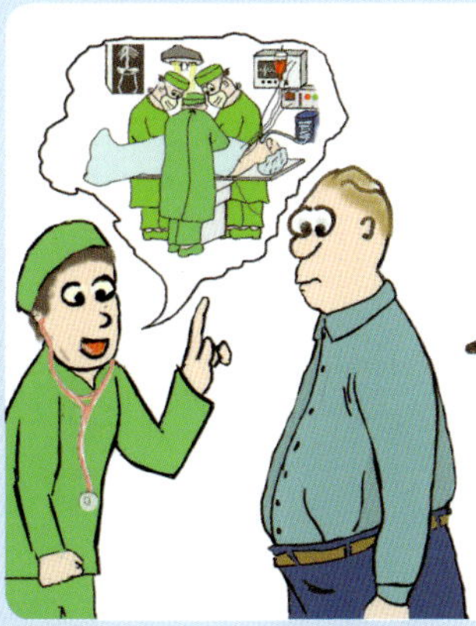

„fasting"	from 10 pm on	don´t drink	don´t eat	don´t smoke
„nüchtern"	ab 22 Uhr	nicht trinken	nicht essen	nicht rauchen
"ناشتا"	از ساعت ۱۰ شب	چیزی نخورید.	چیزی ننوشید.	سیگار نکشید.

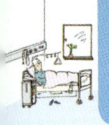

Nursing	Pflege	پرستاری
Clothing	Kleidung	لباس

headscarf / Kopftuch / روسری

handkerchief / Taschentuch / دستمال

glasses – cleaning / Brille – putzen / عینک - تمیزکردن

stick / Stock / عصا

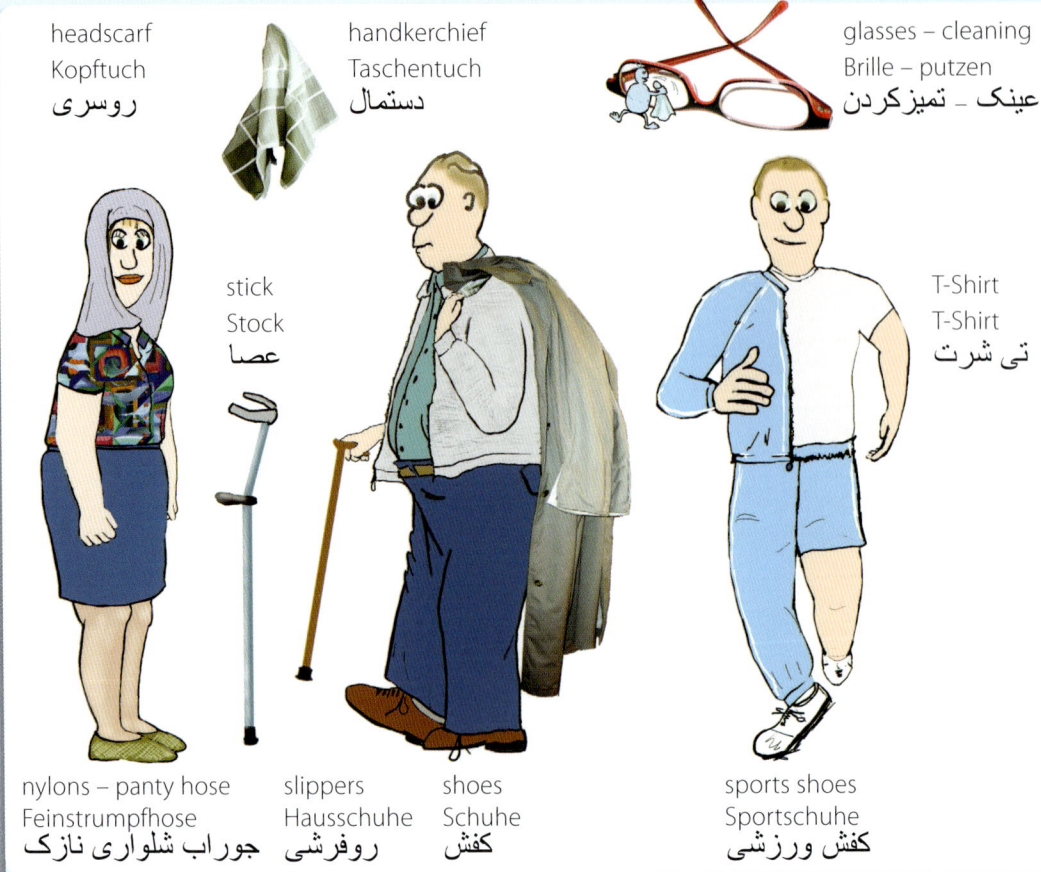

T-Shirt / T-Shirt / تی شرت

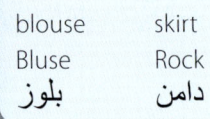

nylons – panty hose / Feinstrumpfhose / جوراب شلواری نازک

slippers / Hausschuhe / روفرشی

shoes / Schuhe / کفش

sports shoes / Sportschuhe / کفش ورزشی

blouse	skirt	shirt	vest	coat	pants	tracksuit
Bluse	Rock	Oberhemd	Weste	Mantel	Hose	Trainingsanzug
بلوز	دامن	پیراهن مردانه	جلیقه	پالتو	شلوار	لباس ورزشی

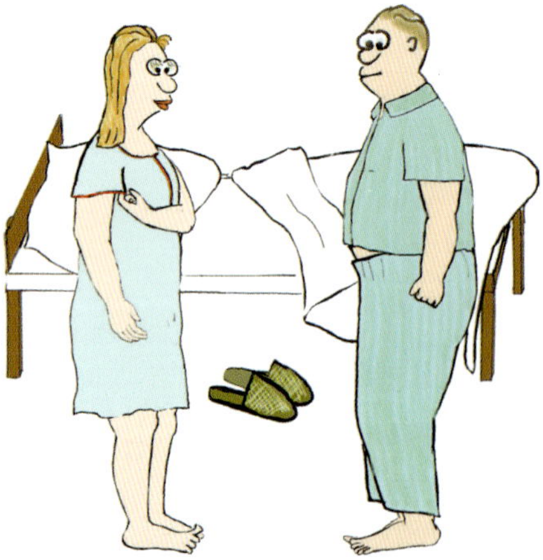

undershirt / Unterhemd / زیرپوش

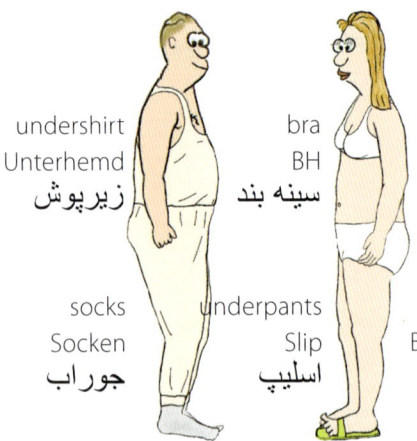

bra / BH / سینه بند

socks / Socken / جوراب

underpants / Slip / اسلیپ

flip-flops / Badelatschen / دمپائی

night dress / Nachthemd / پیراهن خواب

pyjama / Schlafanzug / لباس خواب

underwear / Unterwäsche / لباس زیر

70

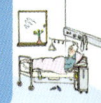

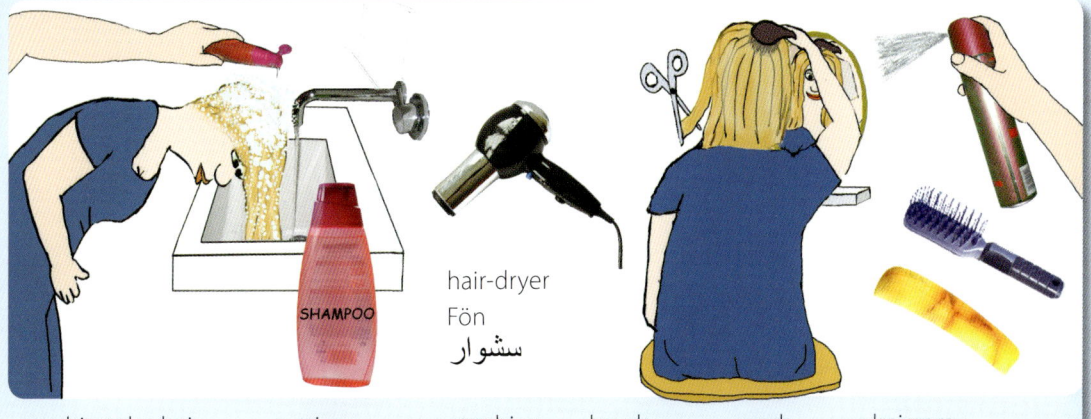

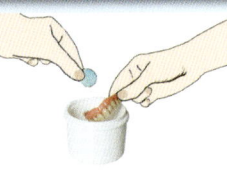

Nursing	**Pflege**	پرستاری
Body care	Körperpflege	نظافت بدن

washing the hair	cutting	combing	brush	comb	hairspray
Haare waschen	schneiden	kämmen	Bürste	Kamm	Haarspray
موها شستن	کوتاه کردن	شانه کردن	برس	شانه	اسپری مو

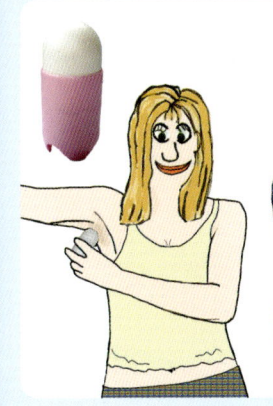

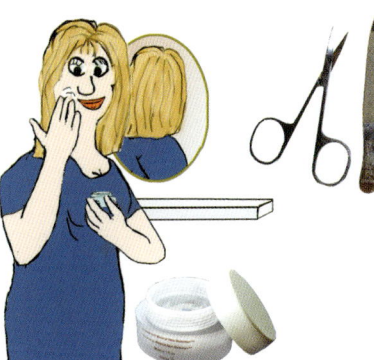

hair-dryer
Fön
سشوار

nail scissors – nail file
Nagelschere – Nagelfeile
ناخن گیر – سوهان ناخن

deo	facial cream	soap/shower gel	body milk
Deo	Gesichtscreme	Seife/Duschgel	Körpermilch
عطر	کرم صورت	صابون / شامپو	کرم بدن

denture cleaner
Prothesenreinigung
تمیز کردن پروتز

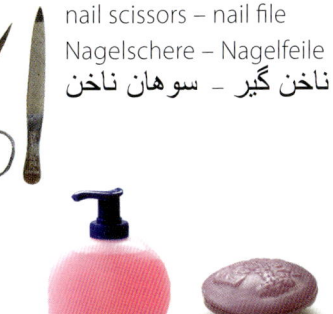

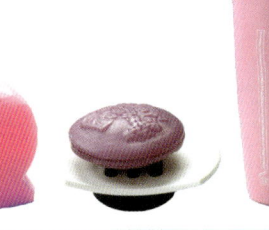

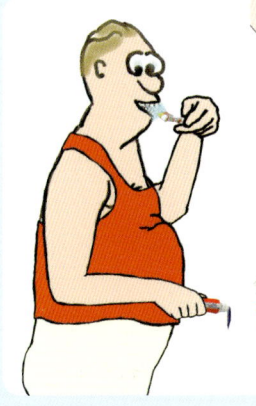

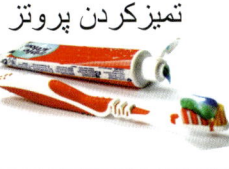

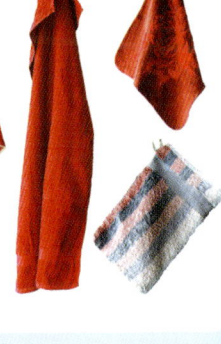

brushing the teeth	tooth paste	shave	towel	washrag
Zähne putzen	Zahnpasta	rasieren	Handtuch	Waschlappen
مسواک زدن دندان	خمیر دندان	تراشیدن ریش	حوله	لیف حمام

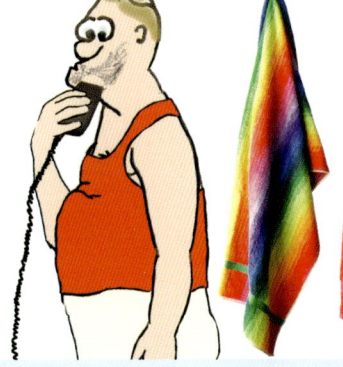

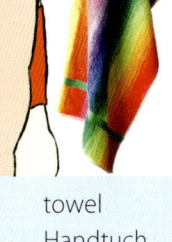

71

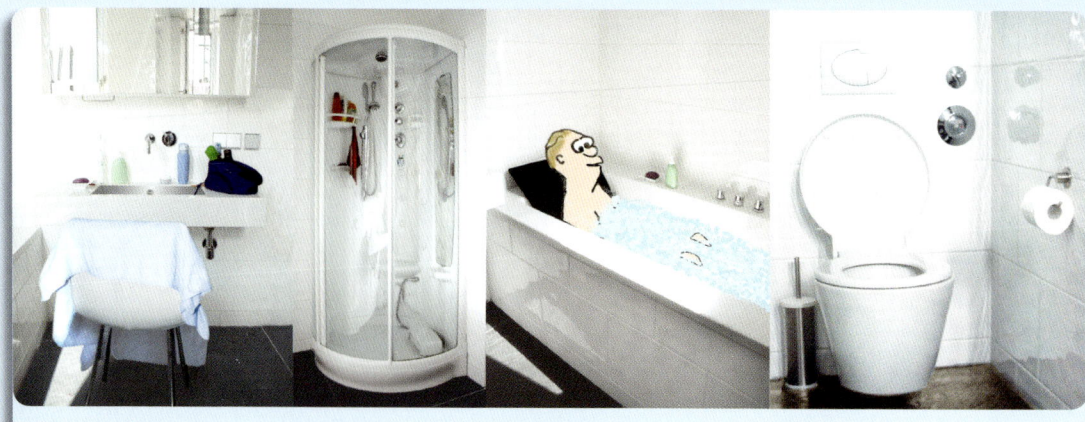

Nursing
Body care

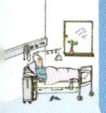

Pflege
Körperpflege

پرستاری
نظافت بدن

to the washbasin	shower	into the bathtub	to the toilet
ans Waschbecken	duschen	in die Wanne	auf die Toilette
جلوی دستشوئی	دوش گرفتن	در وان	در توالت

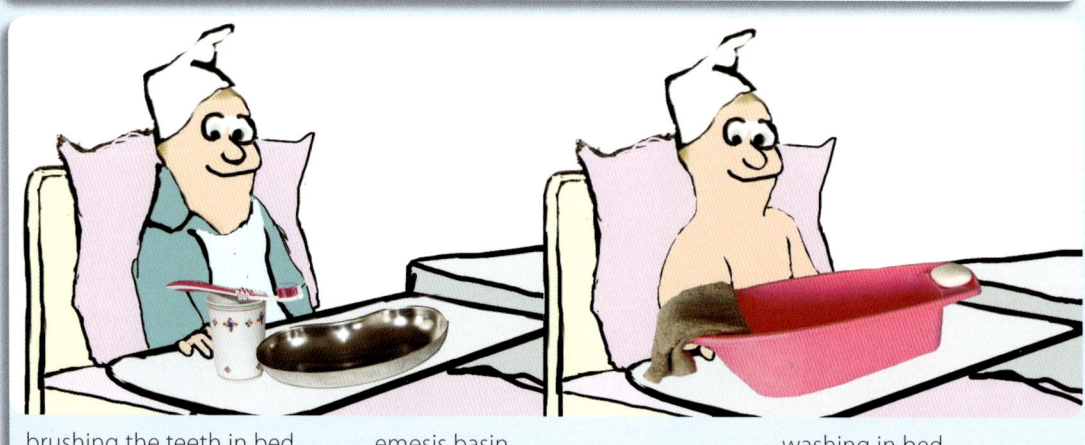

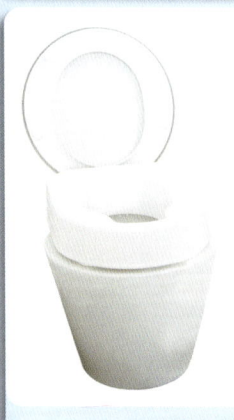

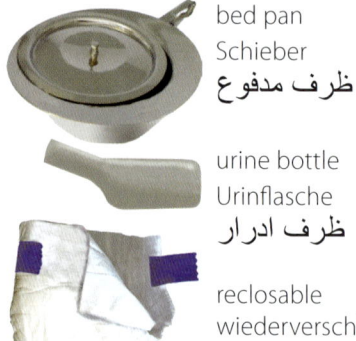

brushing the teeth in bed	emesis basin	washing in bed
Zähne putzen im Bett	Nierenschale	Waschen im Bett
مسواک زدن در تخت خواب	کاسه بیمارستان	شستن در تخت خواب

bed pan
Schieber
ظرف مدفوع

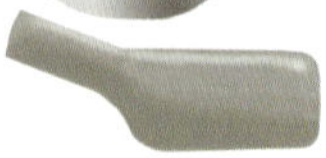

urine bottle
Urinflasche
ظرف ادرار

reclosable
wiederverschließbar
با قابلیت بستن دوباره

toilet booster seat	commode	diapers
Toilettensitzerhöhung	Nachtstuhl/WC-Stuhl	Windeln
بالا بردن توالت	صندلی توالت	پوشک کردن

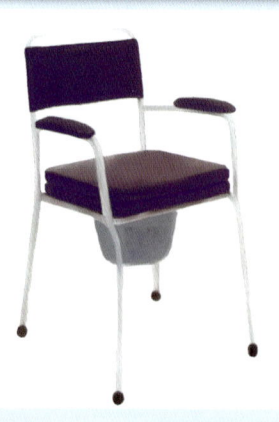

72

Nursing / Pflege
Bedding / Betten

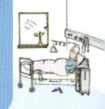

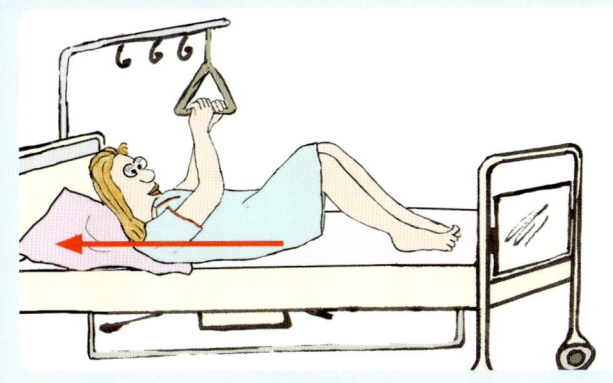

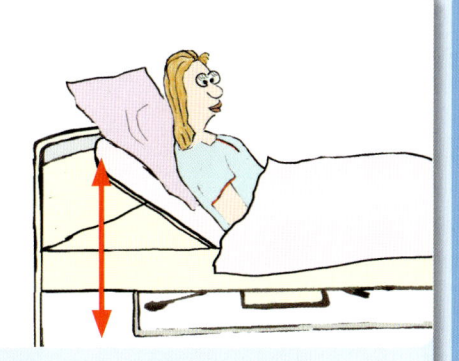

پرستاری
در تختخواب

sliding up in bed: bend your knees – head to chest – push off
im Bett hochrutschen: Beine anziehen – Kopf auf die Brust – abstoßen
در تختخواب به طرف بالا رفتن: زانوها را جمع کنید. ـ سر به طرف جلو ـ فشار به طرف بالا

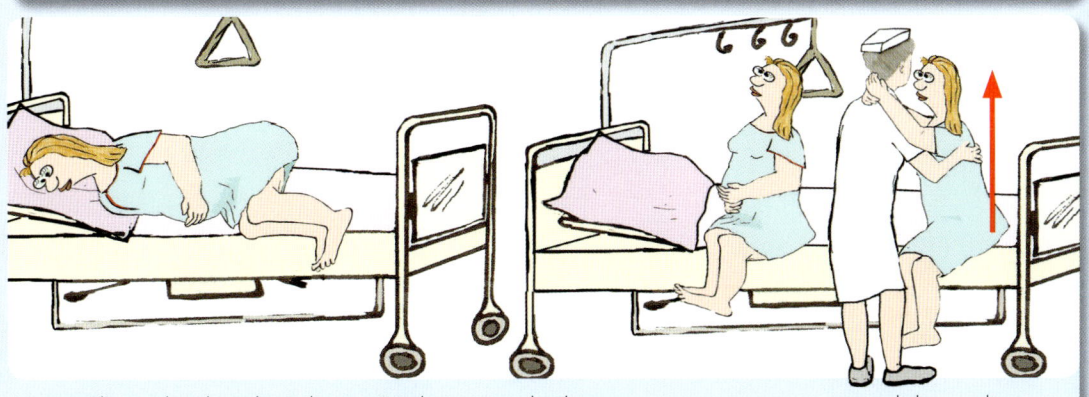

higher – lower
höher – tiefer
بالاتر ـ پائین تر

turn sidewards – hand on the stomach
auf die Seite drehen – Hand auf den Bauch
به پهلو بخوابید. ـ دست را روی شکم بگذارید.

look up
hochgucken
به سمت بالا نگاه کنید.

arm around the neck
Arme um den Hals
دستها را دور گلو حلقه کنید.

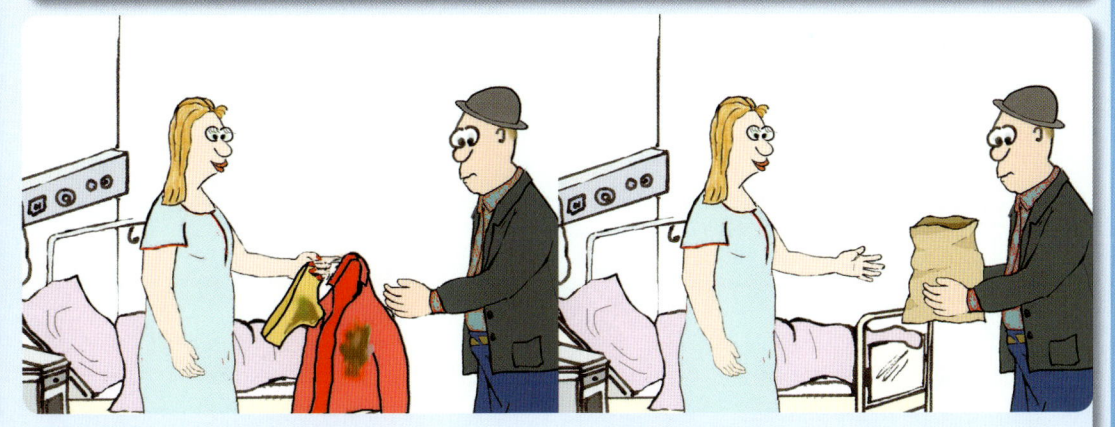

visitors should take along …
Besuch soll mitnehmen …
مهمان باید … را با خود ببرد.

… bring along
… mitbringen
… را با خود بیاورد.

Nursing
Condition/eating

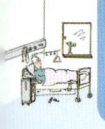

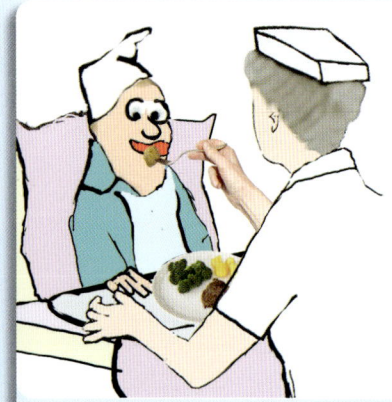

Pflege
Befinden/Essen

پرستاری
نظر دادن / غذا خوردن

spoon-feeding	cold	warm	wheelchair	walker
Essen reichen – füttern	kalt	heiß	Rollstuhl	Rollator
غذا دادن	سرد	گرم	صندلی چرخدار	عصای چرخدار

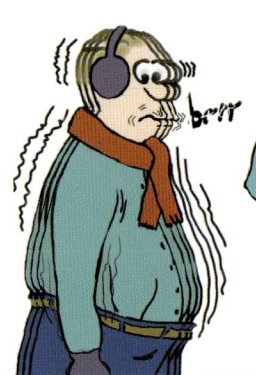

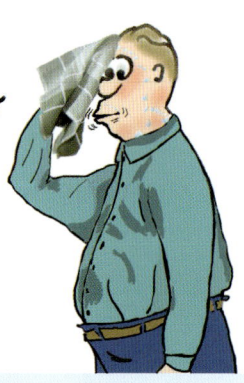

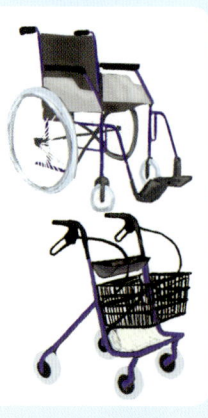

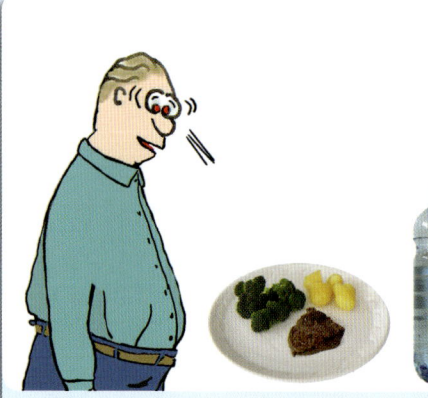

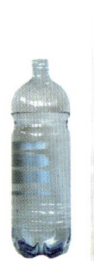

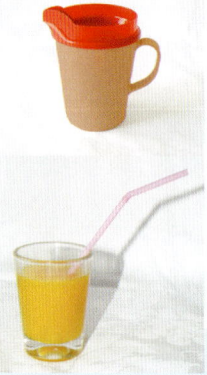

hunger	thirst	spout cup – straw	at the table
Hunger	Durst	Schnabeltasse – Strohhalm	an den Tisch
گرسنگی	تشنگی	لیوان نوکدار - نی	سر میز

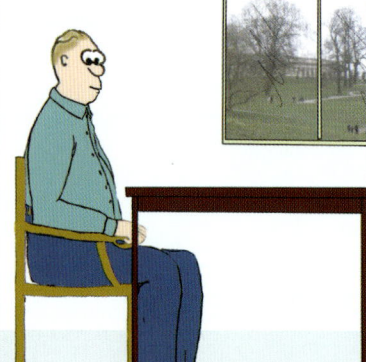

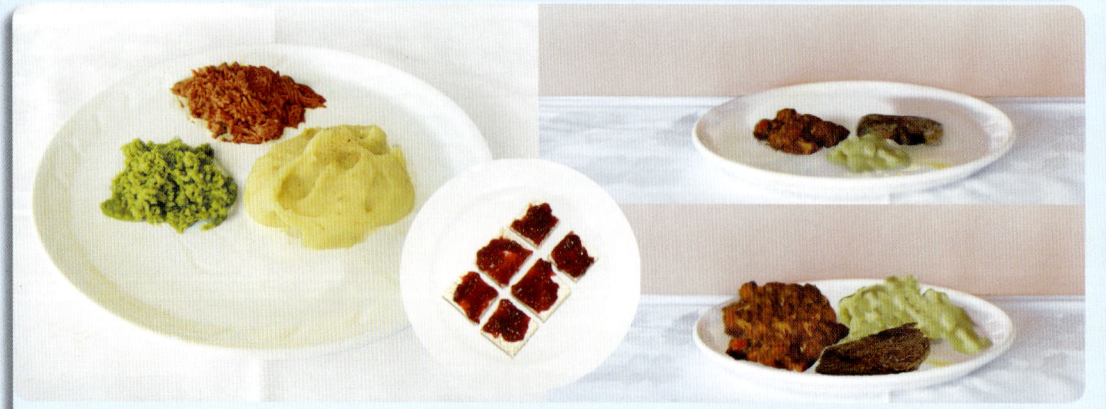

pureed diet	in small bits – morsel	small portion	large portion
passierte Kost	Häppchen	kleine Portion	große Portion
غذای آماده	لقمه	پُرس کوچک	پُرس بزرگ

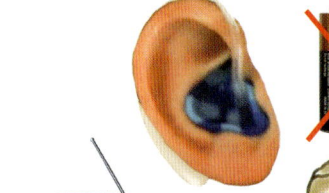

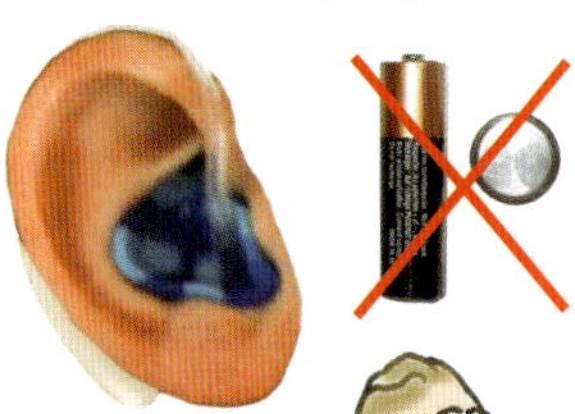

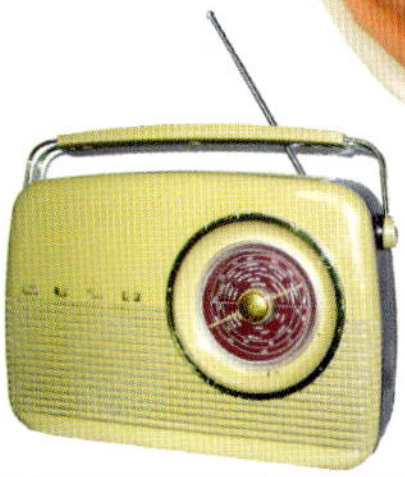

Nursing
Activities/religion

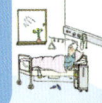

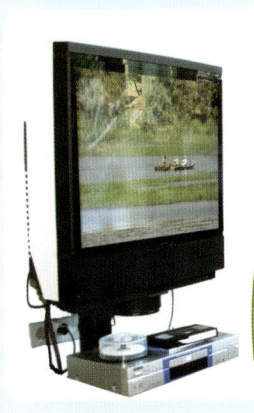

Pflege
Aktivitäten/Religion

پرستاری
فعالیتها / دین

hearing aid – batteries empty
Hörgerät – Batterien leer
سمعک - باطری ندارد.

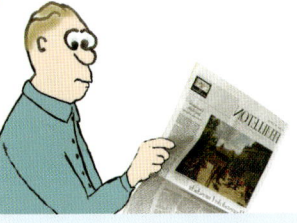

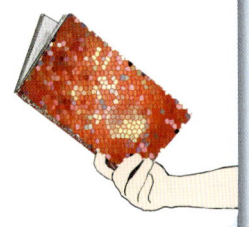

watching TV	listening to the radio	reading a newspaper	reading a book
fernsehen	Radio hören	Zeitung lesen	Buch lesen
تلویزیون دیدن	رادیو گوش کردن	روزنامه خواندن	کتاب خواندن

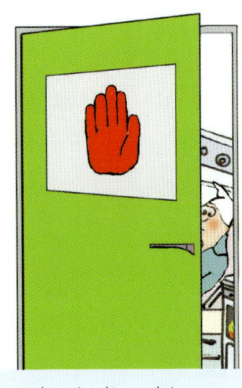

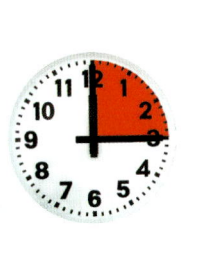

Please don´t disturb!
Bitte nicht stören!
لطفا مزاحم نشویید!

floating water – pitcher
fließendes Wasser/Krug – Kanne
آب روان / تُنگ - قوری

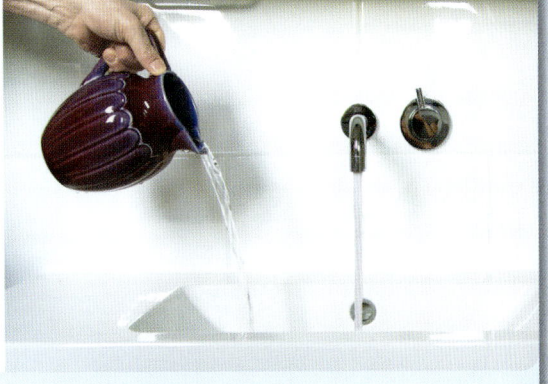

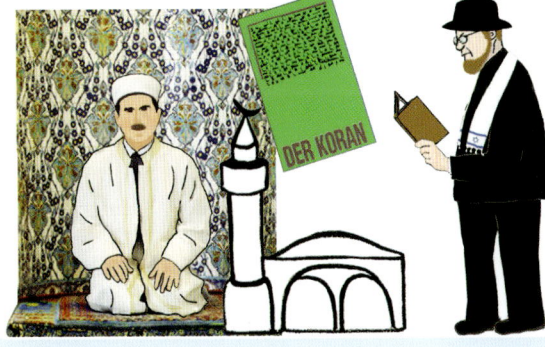

talk to an imam	to the mosque	rabbi	to church	talk to a priest
Imam sprechen	in die Moschee	Rabbi	in die Kirche	Priester sprechen
با امام جماعت صحبت کردن	به مسجد رفتن	خاخام	به کلیسا رفتن	با کشیش صحبت کردن

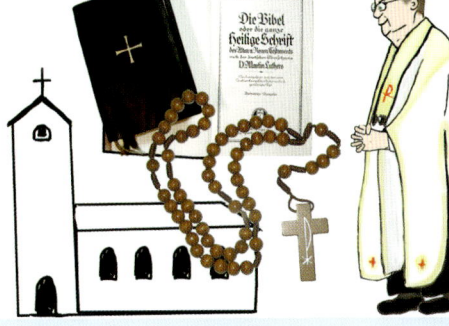

75

In the pharmacy | In der Apotheke | در داروخانه

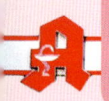

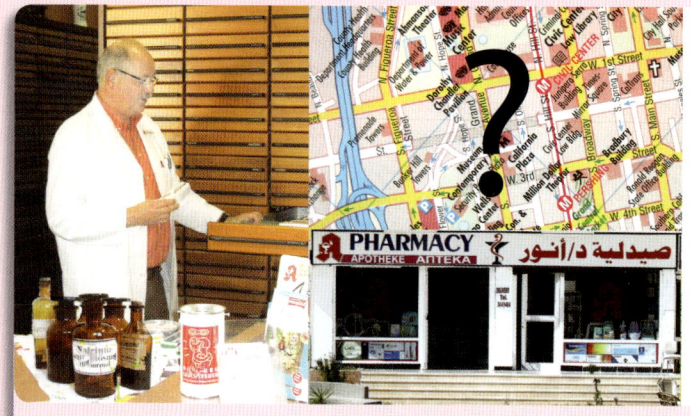

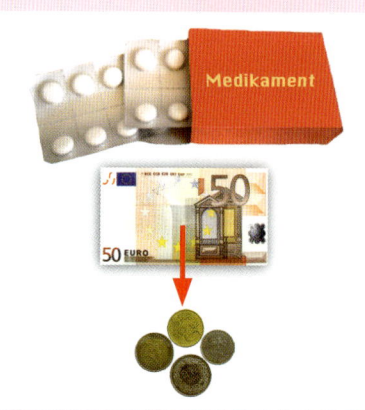

Where is the next pharmacy/chemist´s?
Wo ist die nächste Apotheke?
داروخانه بعدی کجاست؟

Is there a cheaper medicine available?
Gibt es das (Medikament) auch billiger?
این (دارو) ارزانتر هم پیدا میشود؟

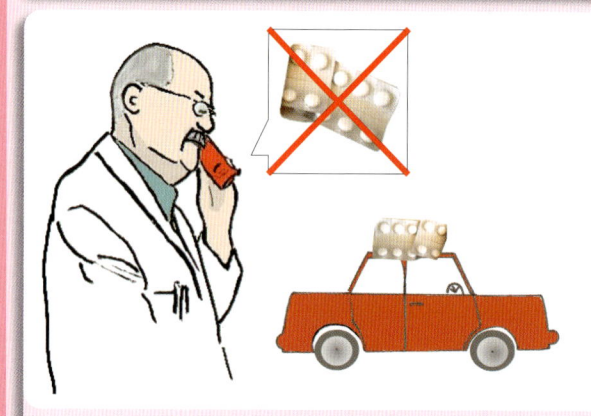

We have to order it first.
Das müssen wir erst bestellen.
ما باید اول این را سفارش دهیم.

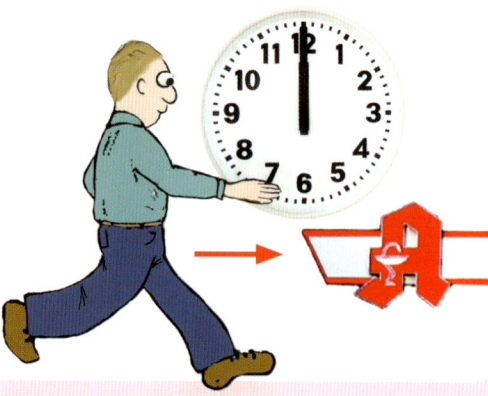

Come back at … clock.
Wiederkommen um … Uhr.
ساعت … دوباره بیائید.

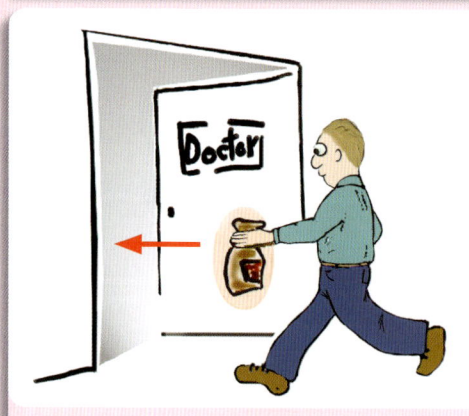

with medicine back to the practice
mit dem Medikament in die Praxis
با دارو به مطب دکتر بروید.

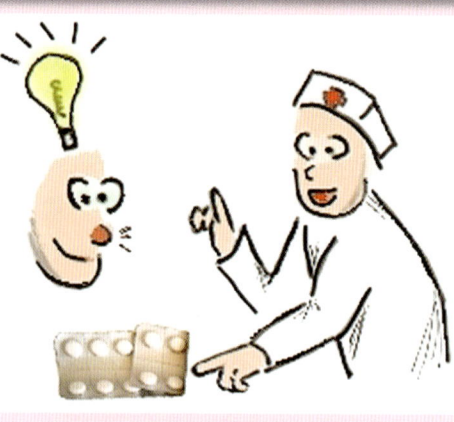

let them show you the application
Anwendung zeigen lassen
روش مصرف را بپرسید.

Traveler´s health kit   Reiseapotheke   داروخانه مسافرت

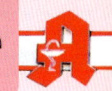

Health insurance coverage
In principle, you should ask your health insurance about their coverage for traveling in foreign countries and overseas.

Traveler´s health kit
in accordance with your physician, according to travel destination, -time und traveling manner

– medication against pain or fever e.g. paracetamol, diclofenac and/or butylscopolamin against cramps
– antidiarrheal medication e.g. loperamide, oral rehydration solution packets, antacid, metoclopramide drops, perenterol-capsules, mild laxative
– antibiotic for self-treatment of severe diarrhea or cystitis
– antihistamine, insect repellent, tick tweezer, mosquito net
– decongestant, cough suppressant/expectorant, thermometer
– sports cream e. g. diclofenac gel
– dressing strip, gauze bandages at 4, 6, 8 cm, ace wraps at 8, 10 cm
– antiseptic, adhesive bandages, scissors, gloves
– personal medicine in their original containers and a copy of the prescription, and if necessary a letter from your physician about your personal medication and injectionrequirements according to the import regulations
– replacement glasses, sunglasses, sunscreen
– condoms, antifungal vaginal suppositories or creams
– compression stockings for long lasting flights

Special questions to your physician
Prevention of malaria, yellow fever-, hepatitis-, meningococcal vaccination?

Der Integrationsbeauftragte der Landesregierung Nordrhein-Westfalen

LEBENSRETTER GESUCHT
Helfen bei der Freiwilligen Feuerwehr

Abdelwahed Ibanayaden, Freiwillige Feuerwehr Siegen | Taci Simsek, Berufsfeuerwehr Krefeld | Mehmet Arif Aslan, Berufsfeuerwehr Dortmund | Fatih Bayrak, Freiwillige Feuerwehr Meschede

www.integrationsbeauftragter.nrw.de

Bundesamt für Migration und Flüchtlinge

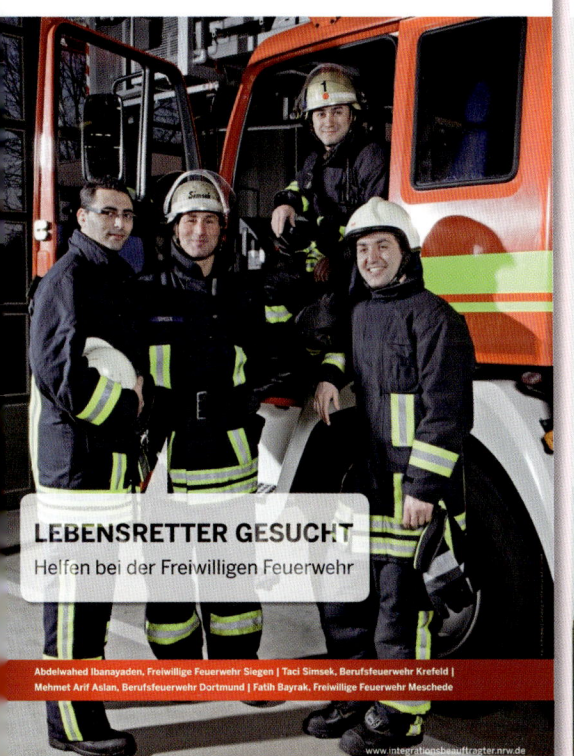

Informationen zum Thema Integration

Was ist ein Integrationskurs?
Wo finden Migranten Hilfe und Ansprechpartner?
Diese und viele weitere Fragen beantwortet das Internetportal Integration des Bundesamtes für Migration und Flüchtlinge unter der Adresse:

www.integration-in-deutschland.de

Die zentrale Informationsplattform zum Thema Integration richtet sich an Zuwanderer, interessierte Bürger und Akteure der Integrationsarbeit.

Sie ist anschaulich gestaltet, leicht verständlich und bietet umfassende Informationen in den Sprachen Deutsch, Englisch, Russisch und Türkisch.

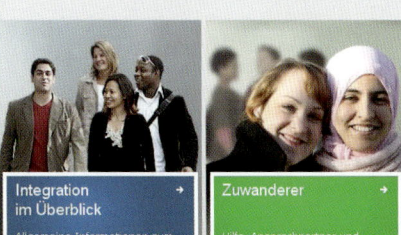

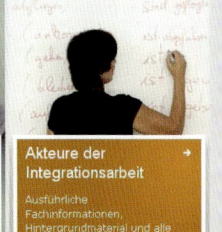

Integration im Überblick →
Allgemeine Informationen zum Thema Integration und Tipps zum Weiterlesen

Zuwanderer →
Hilfe, Ansprechpartner und leicht verständliche Antworten auf die häufigsten Fragen

Akteure der Integrationsarbeit →
Ausführliche Fachinformationen, Hintergrundmaterial und alle wichtigen Formulare

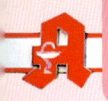

Traveler's health kit — Reiseapotheke — داروخانه مسافرت

Krankenversicherungsschutz
Man sollte sich grundsätzlich vor jeder Auslandsreise bei seiner Krankenversicherung nach dem Auslandskrankenversicherungsschutz erkundigen.

Reiseapotheke
in Absprache mit dem Hausarzt/in Abhängigkeit von Reiseziel, -dauer und Reiseart

- Mittel gegen einfache Schmerzen und Fieber wie Paracetamol, Diclofenac und/oder Butylscopolamin gegen Krämpfe
- Magen-/Durchfallmittel: Loperamid, Elektrolyt-Lösungen, Metoclopramid-Tropfen, Perenterol-Kapseln, leichtes Abführmittel
- Antibiotikum gegen schwere Diarrhoe oder Blasenentzündung
- Antihistaminikum, Mückenspray, Zeckenzange, Moskitonetz
- Nasenspray, Hustensaft, Fieberthermometer
- Sportsalbe wie Diclofenac Gel
- Wundpflaster, je 1 Mullbinde 4, 6, 8 cm, elastische Binde je 8, 10 cm
- Hautdesinfektion, Heftpflaster, kleine Schere, Handschuhe
- eigene Dauermedikamente in der Originalpackung und mit Rezeptkopie resp. Attest vom Hausarzt über den persönlichen Medikamenten- und Spritzenbedarf entsprechend der Einfuhrbestimmungen
- Ersatzbrille, Sonnenbrille, Sonnenschutzmittel
- Kondome, Scheidenpilzsalbe/-zäpfchen
- Stützstrümpfe bei längeren Flugreisen

Spezielle Fragen an den Hausarzt
Malariaprophylaxe, Gelbfieberimpfung, Hepatitisimpfung, Meningokokken?

بیمه خدمات درمانی
قبل از سفرهای خارجی هرکس باید در مورد بیمه خدمات درمانی خارج از کشور تحقیق کند.

داروخانه مسافرت
با توافق پزشک خانواده / بسته به مقصد، مدت سفر و وسیله سفر

- دارو برای دردهای معمولی و تب مثل پاراسٍتامول، دیکلوفناک ویا بوتیسکوپولامین برای گرفتگی عضلات
- داروی معده / ضد اسهال : لوپرامید، محلول الکترولیت، قطره متوکلوپرامید قرص پرنترول: داروی روان کننده
- آنتی بیوتیک برای اسهال یا عفونت مثانه
- آنتی هیستامین، حشره کُش، موچین برای درآوردن کنه، پشه بند
- اسپری دماغ ، شربت سینه، درجه تب
- پماد مثل کرم دیکلوفناک
- چسب زخم معمولی به ابعاد ۶،٤ ، ۸، کشی ۸ ، ۱۰ سانتی متر
- ضدعفونی کننده، نوار چسب زخم، قیچی کوچک، دستکش
- تعدادی داروی ضروری درجعبه اصلی به همراه کپی نسخه پزشک با گواهی پزشک از خانواده در مورد داروهای شخصی و آمپولهای ضروری مطابق مقررات گمرکی
- عینک اضافی، عینک آفتابی، کرم ضد آفتاب
- کآندوم، کرم ضد قارچ / شیاف آلت تناسلی خانمها
- جوراب شلواری ارتوپدی برای پروازهای طولانی

سوالهای ویژه از پزشک خانواده
پیشگیری از بیماری مالاریا، واکسن تب زرد، واکسن هپاتیت، منینگوکوکن؟

Websites about travel medicine • Internetadressen zur Reisemedizin • آدرسهای اینترنتی داروخانه مسافرت
www.rki.de; www.crm.de (–> Gelbfieber-Impfstelle)
www.bmgfj.gv.at (Gesundheit –> Gesundheitsförderung –> Impfen –> Gelbfieberimpfstellen)
www.bag.admin.ch/themen/medizin (–> Infektionskrankheiten –> Impfungen –> Reisemedizin)
www.fit-for-travel.de; www.dtg.org; wwwn.cdc.gov/travel/contentYellowBook.aspx
www.healthinfotranslations.com

فهرست کلمات کلیدی

کلیه 11U
مثانه 11U
غده پروستات
2U، 8U، 11U
خواب 12
سردرد 14
پیشگیری 25
دفترچه حاملگی 25
دفترچه واکسن 25
تب A، 12، 27
عرق ریختن 12، 33
قرصها 56-58
دارو 56-58
شیر 66
فیلمبرداری مثانه 8U
سوالهای معمول A
شدت درد A
عددها B
پیشگیری
19، 20، 32، 51، U2
آبریزش بینی 12، 27
آپاندیس 23، 31
آرتروز 45
آرزوی بچه 35، 4U
آزمایش ادرار 19، 49
آزمایش بافت پروستات8U
آزمایش خون 49
آزمایش ریه 50
آزمایش مدفوع 32، 49، 2U
آسم 17، 31
آفتابی 60
آمادگی بیمار
برای بیهوشی 69
آمپول 46، 56، 5U
احساس خفگی 17
احساس گرمای ناگهانی33
احساسهای بد 13، 43
اختلال در توانایی
جنسی مردان 4U، 5U
استراحت 59
استرس 15
استفاده 59، 62
استفراغ 18، 27، 40
استفراغ کردن 26
اسهال 19، 28
اشعه 54
اعصاب 14، 15
اعضای بد 22، 23
افزایش وزن B، 33
افسردگی 15، 33
التهاب گلو 31
با پیستید 49
بالا آوردن 26
بچه ها 25-31
بخش گوش و
حلق و بینی 20
بدخوابی 15، 25
برونشیت 12، 17، 31
بلند کردن 59
بواسیر 19
بوی بد دهان 20
بی اشتهایی 18
بیمارستان 68، 69
بیماری جنسی 32، 3U

بیماریهای ارثی 25
بیهوشی 16، 29، 69
پائین آوردن رحم 39
پانسمان 61
پرستاری 70-75
پرسشنامه 8، 9
پریود 34
پزشک ارولوژ 2U-11
پزشک همراه کتاب
پزشک خانواده 12-20
پزشک زنان 35-41
پزشک کودکان 25-31
پوشک کردن 28، 72
پوکی استخوان 45
پیشگیری حاملگی 32، 5U
پیشگیری سرطان روده
تخمدان 39
ترشح 32، 3U
تزریق سرم 56
تشنج 14، 29
تشنگی 18، 74
تغذیه 63-67
تلویزیون 30، 75
تنفس 17
توالت 72
توموگرافی 53
توموگرافی هسته ای 53
جوراب کشی 61
چشم 20، 30
چهاردست و پا راه رفتن 29
حالت تهوع 18، 40
حاملگی 40، 41
حرکت 29، 62
حساسیت 12، 52
حساسیت به رادیولوژی 52
حواله 11
خارش 32، 3U
ختنه به دلائل مذهبی 3U
خستگی 15
خلط 17، 49
خون دماغ 20
خیس کردن جا در خواب 28
داروخانه 76
داروخانه مسافرت 77، 78
در تختخواب 73
درد سیاتیک 45
درد مفصلی 14، 42
درد ناحیه قلبی 16
دردها 13، 14
• سردرد 14
• درد مفصلی 14، 42
• درد ناحیه قلبی 16
• دندان درد 46
• کوفتگی 12
• گلودرد 12، 27
• معده درد 18
درمان 54-62
درمان بوسیله ضربه
موجی 61
دریافت دارو 57، 58

دل پیچه سه ماهه 31
دماغ 20
دندان درد 46
دندانپزشک 46-48
دوران پائینگی 33
دهان 20، 46
دیدن 20، 30
دین 45
دین 75
رادیولوژی سینه 33
راه رفتن 17، 29، 62
رحم 39
رشد 29، 30
روده 19
ریزش مو 33
ریه 33
زایمان زودرس 25
زمانهای B
ژیمناستیک 37، 41، 62
ژیمناستیک درازکش 37، 41، 62، 7U
ژیمناستیک دوران حاملگی 41
ژیمناستیک عضلات پشت 41
ستون فقرات 45
سرایت 12، 27، 31
سرد نگه داشتن 59
سرفه 12، 27
سرماخوردگی 12، 27
سرماخوردگی بهاری 12
سروصدا در گوش 20
سزارین 35
سقط جنین 35
سوزش معده 18
سونوگرافی
• پزشک زنان 33، 41
• لگن 28
• پزشک ارولوژ 2U
• پزشک خانواده 49
سینه 32
شنیدن 20، 30
شیر بدهید 26
صندلی چرخدار 74
ضربان قلب 16
طب سوزنی 60
عدم کنترل ادرار 36، 6U، 7U
عفونت روده 19
عفونت ریه 12، 17، 31
عفونت سقف دهان 12، 31
عفونت گوش میانی 20، 31
عفونت معده- روده 19، 28
عکس رادیولوژی 51-53
عکسبرداری استخوان 51
عمل جراحی 54، 69
غده تیروئید 22، 52
غذا خوردن 63-67، 74
غذا دادن 74
فراموشکاری 15
فشار خون 50
فیلمبرداری معده 51
قارچ 32، 3U
قاشق اندازه گیری 26، 56
قلب 16
کاتد U9
کارت بیمه 11
کامپیوتر 30
کبودی پوست 17
کرمها 19
کشاله ران 23، 44، 11U
کلمه ها 5
کم شنوایی 20، 30، 75
کورتاژ 35

کوفتگی 12
گردش خون 16، 17
گرسنگی 18، 74
گرفتگی عضلات 13، 18، 19، 31، 34
گرفتگی عضلات پا 14
گرم نگه داشتن 29
گلودرد 12، 27
گواهی بیماری 11
گوش 20، 31
گوش درد 20
لثه 39
لباس کف پا 61
لرزش 12، 74
لرزش 15
ماساژ 60
ماساژ با لجن 60
مایعات در گوش میانی 31
متخصص ارتوپدی 42-45
مترجم 55
مدرسه کمردرد 60
مراقبت 8U، 59
مرض قند 67
معاینه 49-53
معاینه روده با دوربین 51
معده 18
معده درد 18
مفصلهای لگن 28، 45
مینیسک زانو 45
میوم 39
ناشتا 46، 69
نبض 50
نسخه 11
نظافت بدن 71، 72
نفخ 19، 31
نوار قلب 50
واریس 17
واکسیناسیون 27
وزن کم کنید B، 59
هضم غذا 19، 28
هنگام پذیرش 11
هنگام نیاز 58
یبوست 19، 28

Index

abdominal cramping 13, 18, 19, 31, 34
abdominal pain 34, 40
abortion 35
activities 75
acupuncture 60
allergy 12, 52
anesthesia 69
appendicitis 23, 31
application 57, 58
appointment 11
arteriosclerosis 17
arthrosis 45
ASS 55
asthma 17, 31

baby 25-31
baby nutrition 26
bedding 73
bedrest 59
bedwetting 28
birth control 32
blood on the stool 19
blood pressure 50
blood sample 49
body care 71, 72
bowel cancer prevention 19, 51
bowles 19
breast feeding 26
breath, bad 20
breathing 17
bronchitis 12, 17, 31
bruises 17

catheter U9
certificate of vaccination 25
cesarean 35
check-up 19, 20, 32, 51, 54
children 25-31
• graphic chart 31
circulation 16, 17
circumcision U3
clothing 70
cold 12, 27
colonoscopy 51
computer 30
computer-tomography 53
concentration 15, 30
constipation 19, 28
contraception 32
contrast media 52
cooling 59
cough 12, 27
cramps in the legs 14
crawling 29
cystitis 28, 32, U2
cystoskopy U8

dairy products 66
defecation 19, 28
dentist 46-48
depression 15, 33
desire for children 35, U4
development 29, 30
diabetes diet 67
diapers 28, 72
diarrhoea 19, 28
diet 63-67

digestion 19, 28
discharge 32, U3
distance 17
diverticula 19

ear 20, 31
ear nose throat 20
ECG 50
epilepsy 29
examination 49-53
exercise 29, 62
exhaustion 15
eyes 20, 30

fainting 16, 29
family diseases 25
family doctor 12-20
fango 60
FAQ B
fasting 46, 69
fedding 74
fever A, 12, 27
forgetfulness 15

gas 19, 31
gastroenteritis 19, 28
gastroscopy 51
graphic charts 22, 23, 31, 39, 45, U11
• family doctor/organs 22, 23
• gynecologist 39
• pediatrician 31
• orthopedist 45
• urologist U11
groin 23, 44, U11
gymnastics 37, 41, 62
gynecologist 32-41
• graphic chart 39

haemorrhoids 19
hair loss 33
hay-fever 12
headache 14
health insurance card 11
hearing 20, 30
heart 16
heart rhythm 16
heartburn 18
hospital 68, 69
hot flushes 33
hunger 18, 74

if required 58
impotence U4, U5
incontinence 36, U6, U7
increase in weight B, 33
infection 12, 27, 31
inflammation of the middle ear 20, U3
influenza 12, 27
infusion 56
injection 46, 56, U5
inoculation 27
insole 61
intensity of pain A
internal medicine 12-20
interpreter 55
irradiation 54
itching 12, 32, U3

kidney diseases U11

lack of appetite 18
lifting 59
lose weight 59
lung function 50

mammography 33
massage 60
maternity card 25, 40
medicine 54, 56-58
meniscus 45
menopause 33
menstruation cycle 34
metformin 52, 55
miscarriage 35
motor activity 29, 62
mud pack therapy 60
myoma 39

nausea 18, 40
nerves, neurology 14, 15
night sweats 12
nose-bleeding 20
nuclear magnetic resonance 53
numbers B
nursing 70-75
nutrition 26, 63-67, 74

operation 54, 69
organs 22, 23
orthopedist 42-45
• graphic chart 45
osteoporosis 45
ovary 39

pain A, 13, 14
• abdominal pain 13, 18, 19, 31, 34
• earache 20
• headache 14
• heartache 16
• pain in the joints 14, 42
• pain in the limbs 12
• pain of the lower body 34, 40
• sore throat 12
• stomachache 18
• tooth pain 46
pediatrician 25-31
• graphic chart 31
pelvic floor gymnastic 37, 41, 62, U7
penis U3, U11
period 34
pharmacy 76
phimosis U3
phlegm 17, 49
pill 32
pneumonia 12, 17, 31
post natal exercises 41
posture training 60
pre-anesthesia discussion 69
pregnancy 40, 41
prescription 11, 76
preterm delivery 25
prevention card 25
preventive check for breast cancer 32

preventive examination 19, 20, 32, 51, U2
prostate U2, U11
prostate biopsy U8
pseudo croup 31
pulse 50

questionnaire 9

reception 11
referral 11, 55
religion 75
rest 59, U8
ringing in the ears 20
routine check 54

seeing 20, 30
seizure disorder 29
sensitivity 13, 43
sexual intercourse 35, U4, U5
sexual transmitted disease 32, U3
shivering 12, 74
shockwave therapy 61
shortness of breath 17
sick report 11
sickness 18, 27, 40
skeletal scintigraphy 51
skeleton 22, 45
sleeping 15, 25
slipped disk 45
smear test 32, 33
smoking 59
sore throat 12
spasms 13, 14, 18, 19, 29, 31, 34
sperm sample U4
spew 26
spinal column 45
spiral 32
spotting 34
stand up 49
stomach 18
stool sample 19, 49
stress 15
suffocation 17
sun protection 60
surgical hose 61
swallowing 20
sweating 12, 33
swollen ankles 16

tablets 56-58
tapes 61
television 30, 75
testicle diseases U11
thirstyness 18, 74
3-month-gripes 31
thrush 32, U3
thyroid gland 22, 52
times B
toilet 72
tonsillitis 12, 31
traveler's health kit 77, 78
treatment 54-62
trembling 15
trouble hearing 20, 30, 75
twitching 14, 29
tympanic effusion 31

ultrasound
• at the family doctor 49
• at the gynecologist 33, 41
• hip joint 28
• at the urologist U2
unconsciousness 16, 27
urge 36, U2, U6
urine sample 32, 49, U2
urologist
 supplement U2-11
• graphic chart U11
uterine descent 37, U7

varicose veins 17
vertigo 14
visitors 73
vocabulary 5
vomiting 18, 27, 40

walking 17, 29, 62
warmth 59, U9
washing 72
weighing B, 26, 33, 59
wheelchair 74
womb 39
worms 19

x-raying 51-53